Instructor's Guide

to Accompany

Calculating Drug Dosages: An Interactive Approach to Learning Nursing Math

SECOND EDITION

Sandra Luz Martinez de Castillo, RN, MA, EdD

Nursing Instructor
Contra Costa College
San Pablo, California

and

Maryanne Werner-McCullough, RN, MS, MNP

Nursing Instructor
Contra Costa College
San Pablo, California

F. A. Davis Company • Philadelphia

F. A. Davis Company
1915 Arch Street
Philadelphia, PA 19103
www.fadavis.com

ISBN-10:   0-8036-1540-X
ISBN-13:   978-0-8036-1540-3

Printed in the United States of America

Last digit indicates print number: 10 9 8 7 6 5 4 3 2

Publisher, Nursing: Robert G. Martone
Associate Acquisitions Editor: Tom Ciavarella
Design Manager: Carolyn O'Brien

NOTE: Author and publisher have done everything possible to ensure content herein is accurate, current, and in accord with accepted standards at the time of publication, and to secure permission to reproduce drug labels. The reader is advised that information related to drugs, including facsimiles of drug labels, is presented for demonstration purposes only, to illustrate calculation methods. The reader is further advised to refer to current pharmaceutical references for information about drug therapy and always check product information (package inserts) for new information regarding dose and contraindications before administering any drug. Caution is especially urged when using new or infrequently ordered drugs.

A Note to the Instructor

Dear Instructor:

The second edition of *Calculating Drug Dosages: An Interactive Approach to Learning Nursing Math* continues to include the application of critical thinking skills in solving realistic clinical drug dosage problems. This edition features new Focus on Safety exercises, as well as a new section preparing the student for the NCLEX licensure examination. The content has been revised to reflect the latest standards for safe medication administration established by the Institute for Safe Medication Practices (ISMP) and the Joint Commission for Accreditation of Healthcare Organizations (JCAHO).

The three components of the program (the CD-ROM, the Student Workbook, and the Instructor's Guide) present a total learning package to help the student master the essential skills of drug dosage calculations. The program can be used as a self-paced learning tool, as a resource for developing competency, or as an assigned reference for any nursing math course.

The **CD-ROM** consists of 13 modules. Within the modules the student will find:

NEW! ◆ Focus on Safety sections to highlight clinical situations and avoid common errors
NEW! ◆ A Preparation for NCLEX module that provides practice problems based on the format of the NCLEX licensure examination
NEW! ◆ Sections on High Alert Medications that link to information from *Davis' Drug Guide*
NEW! ◆ Updated medication labels, approved abbreviations, and units of measurement
◆ A choice of methods for solving problems (linear ratio and proportion, fractional ratio and proportion, dimensional analysis, and formula method)
◆ Clear presentation of realistic clinical situations requiring calculations
◆ Interactive learning activities and critical thinking word problems
◆ Practice problems, Section Quizzes, a Module Review, and Module Tests that allow the student to print out test results
◆ Learning aids, including a pop-up calculator and a glossary (Module Terms)

The **Student Workbook** has new practice problems for each of the modules and contains:

NEW! ◆ Focus on Safety exercises to promote critical thinking and decision making
NEW! ◆ Updated medication labels and approved abbreviations
NEW! ◆ More practice problems with answers at the end of the workbook
◆ Key points, formulas, and tables of equivalent measurement for each module

The **Instructor's Guide** is designed to assist with additional materials for teaching, including:

NEW! ◆ A Focus on Safety section to stimulate discussion of realistic clinical situations
NEW! ◆ A Preparation for NCLEX section with sample NCLEX format questions
NEW! ◆ An appendix explaining High Alert Medications
◆ A summary of the objectives and content of each module
◆ Worksheets for each topic, ready to be reproduced for student use
◆ A Basic Math Diagnostic Exam and two Comprehensive Competency Exams
◆ Answers to all exams and Module Tests from the CD-ROM

We hope that you find the second edition of *Calculating Drug Dosages: An Interactive Approach to Learning Nursing Math* relevant and useful to you and your students.

Sandra and Maryanne

CONTENTS

Module: BASIC MATH REVIEW

TO THE INSTRUCTOR:
The Basic Math Review Module assists students in reviewing previously learned math concepts, and reinforces basic math calculations using an interactive format. It is recommended that the Basic Math Module be assigned to all students.

<u>Highlights of the module:</u> Basic Math Review covers how to add, subtract, multiply, and divide fractions and decimals. This module also teaches the student how to read and write Roman numerals. The module supports the following objectives:

FRACTIONS

OBJECTIVES:
1. Compare the value of common fractions.
2. Reduce fractions to their lowest terms.
3. Change mixed numbers to fractions.
4. Define lowest common denominator (LCD).
5. Find the LCD for two or more fractions.
6. Add and subtract fractions with the same or different denominators.
7. Change mixed numbers to improper fractions.
8. Add and subtract mixed numbers.
9. Multiply and divide proper and improper fractions.

DECIMALS

OBJECTIVES:
1. Read common decimal numbers.
2. Compare the value of decimal numbers and round decimal numbers.
3. Line up decimals correctly for addition and subtraction.
4. Add and subtract decimal numbers.
5. Multiply and divide decimal numbers.
6. Correctly place the decimal point in the answer after multiplying and dividing decimals.
7. Use the rules of rounding to round to the whole number, the tenths, hundredths, or thousandths place.
8. Use zeros as placeholders in rounding.

ROMAN NUMERALS

OBJECTIVES:
1. Read and write common Roman numerals.
2. State the value of commonly used Roman numerals.
3. State the rules for the addition and subtraction of Roman numerals.
4. Add and subtract common Roman numerals.

Worksheet:
Using Decimals and Fractions in Medication Administration

For extra practice, solve the following problems.

1. The nurse is to give 3/4 of a tablet. Shade in the amount the nurse will give.
   The decimal equivalent of the fraction 3/4 is _____

2. The nurse is to give 1/2 of a tablet. Shade in the amount the nurse will give.
   The decimal equivalent of the fraction 1/2 is _____

3. The nurse is to give 1/4 of a tablet. Shade in the amount the nurse will give.
   The decimal equivalent of the fraction 1/4 is _____

4. The following tablets are given to the patient during the 7 – 3 shift. What is the total number of tablets that the day nurse gave the patient during the shift? _____

MEDICATION	AMOUNT	TIME GIVEN
Digoxin 0.25 mg p.o. once a day	tabs 1/2	[9:00 AM]
KCl 30 mEq p.o. daily	tabs 1 1/2	[10:00 AM]
Furosemide 20 mg p.o. once a day	tabs 1/2	[10:00 AM]
Levothyroxine 0.1 mg p.o. once a day	tabs 1	[10:00 AM]
Hydralazine 15 mg p.o. once a day	tabs 1.5	[10:00 AM]
Meperidine 50 mg p.o. q.3h. p.r.n. pain	tabs 1	[7:30 AM and 2:00 PM]
Meperidine 100 mg p.o. q.3h. p.r.n. pain	tabs 2	[10:30 AM]

5. The doctor orders 0.65 g of a medication. The pharmacy sends the following: one bottle of tablets labeled 0.225 g per tablet and another bottle labeled 0.2 g per tablet.

   If the nurse gives one tablet from each bottle, the patient will receive _____ g. To give the ordered dose, the nurse must give ___tablet(s) of 0.225 g and ____tablets(s) of 0.2 g.

6. The doctor orders 7.5 mg of a medication. The pharmacy sends the following: one bottle of capsules labeled 3 mg per capsule and another bottle labeled 1.5 mg per capsule.

   If the nurse gives one capsule from each bottle, the patient will receive _____ mg.
   To give the ordered dose, the nurse must give ___ of the 3 mg capsules(s) and ____ of the 1.5 mg capsules(s).

Name: _____

Date: _____

Worksheet:
Using Decimals in Medication Administration

For extra practice, use the Physician's Orders and the Drug Label to solve the following problems.

To solve the problems, divide the ordered amount from the Physician's Orders by the amount found on the **Drug Label.**

1.

Date	Physician's Orders
7/24	**Give 0.5 of Drug A.**
	Patient's name ID *******

Drug Label

Drug A 0.25

The calculated dose is:

_____

2.

Date	Physician's Orders
7/24	**Give 0.125 of Drug B.**
	Patient's name ID *******

Drug Label

Drug B 0.5

The calculated dose is:

_____

3.

Date	Physician's Orders
7/24	**Give 2.25 of Drug C.**
	Patient's name ID *******

Drug Label

Drug C 4.5

The calculated dose is:

_____

4.

Date	Physician's Orders
7/24	**Give 150 of Drug D.**
	Patient's name ID *******

Drug Label

Drug D 1.2

The calculated dose is:

_____

5.

Date	Physician's Orders
7/24	**Give 6.25 of Drug E.**
	Patient's name ID *******

Drug Label

Drug E 25

The calculated dose is:

_____

Date: _____

Worksheet:
Rounding Decimals in Medication Administration

For extra practice, solve the following problems.

1. After calculating a drug dose, the nurse arrives at 1.67777 mL as the answer. The nurse is instructed to round the answer to the <u>thousandths place</u>. The nurse will give _____ mL of the drug.

2. After calculating a drug dose, the nurse arrives at 1.67777 mL as the answer. The nurse is instructed to round the answer to the <u>hundredths</u> place. The nurse will give _____ mL of the drug.

3. After calculating a drug dose, the nurse arrives at 1.67777 mL as the answer. The nurse is instructed to round the answer to the <u>tenths</u> place. The nurse will give _____ mL of the drug.

4. After calculating a drug dose, the nurse arrives at 1.67777 mL as the answer. The nurse is instructed to round the answer to a <u>whole number</u>. The nurse will give _____ mL of the drug.

5. After calculating a drug dose, the nurse arrives at 2.43333 mL as the answer. The nurse is instructed to round the answer to the <u>thousandths place</u>. The nurse will give _____ mL of the drug.

6. After calculating a drug dose, the nurse arrives at 2.43333 mL as the answer. The nurse is instructed to round the answer to the <u>hundredths place</u>. The nurse will give _____ mL of the drug.

7. After calculating a drug dose, the nurse arrives at 2.43333 mL as the answer. The nurse is instructed to round the answer to the <u>tenths place</u>. The nurse will give _____ mL of the drug.

8. After calculating a drug dose, the nurse arrives at 2.43333 mL as the answer. The nurse is instructed to round the answer to a <u>whole number</u>. The nurse will give _____ mL of the drug.

9. After calculating a drug dose, the nurse arrives at 0.45 mL as the answer. The nurse is instructed to round the answer to the <u>tenths place</u>. The nurse will give _____ mL of the drug.

10. After calculating a drug dose, the nurse arrives at 1.84 mL as the answer. The nurse is instructed to round the answer to a <u>whole number</u>. The nurse will give _____ mL of the drug.

Worksheet:
Using Roman Numerals

1. For each of the Roman numerals listed below, write the equivalent arabic number.

   a. i = _____   b. v = _____   c. x = _____   d. iv = _____

   e. vi = _____   f. ix = _____   g. xii = _____   h. iii = _____

2. The nurse is recording the following amounts of liquid taken by the patient during the shift. For each quantity, write the equivalent arabic number.

Patient Intake		Patient Intake:
7/24		
	0800 – oz vii	_____ oz
	0930 – tsp ii	_____ tsp
	1000 – Tbs vi	_____ Tbs
	Patient's name ID ********	

Patient Intake		Patient Intake:
9/13		
	1215 – oz xxv	_____ oz
	1300 – tsp xv	_____ tsp
	1430 – Tbs iv	_____ Tbs
	Patient's name ID ********	

3. A patient record lists the following quantities of medication. For each quantity, write the equivalent Roman numeral.

   a. 41 oz = oz _____   b. 3 tsp = tsp _____   c. 1 T   = T _____

   d. 50 mL = mL _____   e. 30 mL = mL _____   f. 19 mL = mL _____

4. The following quantities of medication are listed on a medication administration record. Look at each quantity and apply the rules for writing Roman numerals.

Medication Record	
3/4	a. Give 90 mL
	b. Give 30 oz
	c. Give 100 mL
	d. Give 15 oz
	Patient's name ID ********

Rewrite the quantities according to the rules for writing Roman numerals.

Medication Record	
3/4	a. Give _____
	b. Give _____
	c. Give _____
	d. Give _____
	Patient's name ID ********

Module: METHODS OF CALCULATION

TO THE INSTRUCTOR:

The Methods of Calculation Module teaches four different methods of calculating drug dosages: linear ratio and proportion, fractional ratio and proportion, dimensional analysis, and the formula method. Unifying concepts (such as the dosage strength, the medication order, and matching the units of measurement) are covered for each method.

<u>Highlights of the module:</u> Methods of Calculation introduces the student to dosage calculations, and then allows the student to choose among the common methods of solving drug dosage problems. Practice in solving simple drug dosage problems is included. The module supports the following objectives:

LINEAR AND FRACTIONAL RATIO AND PROPORTION

OBJECTIVES:
1. Define ratio and proportion.
2. Set up a ratio and proportion using the linear and fractional formats.
3. Identify the known and unknown ratios in a proportion.
4. Write linear or fractional proportions.
5. Solve drug dosage calculation problems using the linear or fractional ratio and proportion method.

DIMENSIONAL ANALYSIS

OBJECTIVES:
1. Describe the dimensional analysis method of calculation.
2. Define conversion factor.
3. Discuss dosage strength as a conversion factor.
4. Set up a problem using dimensional analysis.
5. Select appropriate conversion factors for dimensional analysis problems.
6. Solve drug dosage calculation problems using dimensional analysis.

THE FORMULA METHOD

OBJECTIVES:
1. Define D, H, and V.
2. Identify D, H, and V in a word problem.
3. Correctly place D, H, and V to set up the formula.
4. Write D, H, and V in the formula.
5. Solve drug dosage calculation problems using the formula method.

Worksheet:
Methods of Calculation

For extra practice, solve the following problems.

1. The medication administration record has the following medications listed:
   a. Lanoxin 0.25 mg p.o. daily.   [2200]
   b. KCl 30 mEq p.o. daily.   [1000]
   c. Furosemide 20 mg p.o. b.i.d.   [1000 - 2200]
   d. Enalapril 1.25 mg p.o. b.i.d.   [1000 - 2200]
   e. Ibuprofen 400 mg p.o. q.4h. p.r.n. pain.

   a. At 2130, the nurse answered the patient's call light. The patient was complaining of arthritis pain. The medication record states that the patient received ibuprofen 400 mg at 1830 for pain. The nurse finds the following medications in the medication drawer. Circle the medications that the nurse will give to the patient at 2200.

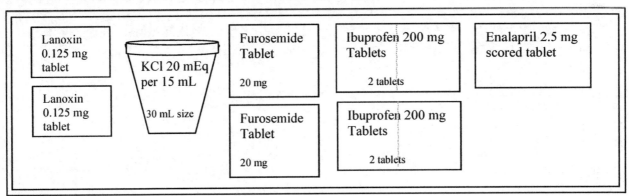

   b. How many tablets of enalapril will the nurse administer at 2200? _____

   c. How many mL of the KCl will the nurse administer at 1000? _____

2. The order is for heparin sodium 2000 units subcut now. The nurse has the following medication in the medication cart. How many mL will the nurse administer?

   Heparin Sodium

   5000 units per mL

   _____

3.a. The doctor orders amoxicillin 500 mg q.8h. for the patient. The pharmacy sends the following medication. Is this the correct medication?

_____

```
┌─────────────────────┐
│ ┌─────────────────┐ │
│ │  Amoxicillin    │ │
│ │ Chewable Tablets│ │
│ │                 │ │
│ │ 125 mg / tablet │ │
│ └─────────────────┘ │
└─────────────────────┘
```

b. How many tablets will the nurse administer to the patient?

_____

4. The order is for oral morphine solution 30 mg q.3h. around the clock. Oral morphine solution is available in 20 mg / 5 mL. How many mL will the patient receive?

_____

5. The order is for aluminum hydroxide 20 mL p.o. q.i.d. The pharmacy sends the following medication. How many mg will the patient receive per dose?

_____

```
    Aluminum
    hydroxide
    320 mg
    per 5 mL
```

6. The doctor orders medroxyprogesterone injection 150 mg IM. The nurse has the following 2.5 mL vial of medroxyprogesterone. How many mL will the nurse administer to the patient?

```
┌───────────────────────────┐
│ 2.5 mL vial               │
│                           │
│ MEDROXYPROGESTERONE       │
│     For injection         │
│   400 mg / mL             │
└───────────────────────────┘
```

_____

7. The emergency room nurse is preparing to give phenytoin 60 mg IV. The drug is available in a 2 mL ampule labeled 50 mg / mL. How many mL will the nurse draw up into the syringe?

_____

8. The medication administration record has the following medications listed:

7/14 1. Dyphylline 150 mg p.o. q.8h.	[0800 – 1600 - 0000]
2. Cefaclor 500 mg p.o. q.8h.	[0800 – 1600 - 0000]
3. Start tapering prednisone as follows:	
Prednisone 15 mg p.o. b.i.d. Start 7/14	[0800 - 2000]
Prednisone 10 mg p.o. b.i.d. Start 7/16	[0800 - 2000]
Prednisone 10 mg p.o. daily Start 7/18	[0800]
Prednisone 5 mg p.o. daily Start 7/20	[0800]
Prednisone 5 mg p.o. every other day Start 7/23	[0800]
4. Guaifenesin 350 mg p.o. q.4h. p.r.n. cough	

a. At 0745 on 7/16, the patient puts on the call light and requests cough syrup. The nurse checks the medication administration record, and the patient has not had any cough syrup overnight. In the medicine drawer below, circle the medications that the nurse will bring in to the patient at 0800.

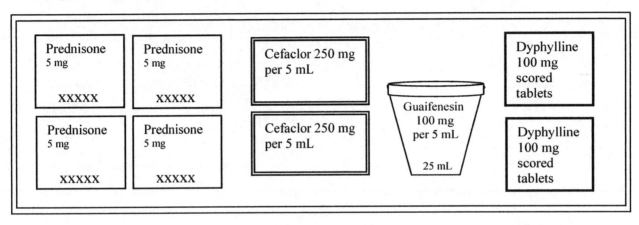

b. How many mL of guaifenesin cough syrup will the nurse give to the patient?

_____

c. How many dyphylline tablets will the nurse give at 0800?

_____

d. How many mg of prednisone will the patient be given at 0800 on 7/24?

_____

9. The doctor orders 375 mg of an oral medication for the patient. The drug is available in a solution that contains 125 mg per 5 mL. How many mL will the nurse administer?

_____

10. The patient is to receive 0.5 g of an antibiotic syrup. The pharmacy sends a bottle of the syrup labeled 1 g / 0.5 mL. How many mL will the nurse administer?

_____

Module: SYSTEMS OF MEASUREMENT

TO THE INSTRUCTOR:
The Systems of Measurement Module teaches the metric and household systems of measurement. The students will work with various units of measurement and learn how each system of measurement is used in clinical practice.

<u>Highlights of the module</u>: Systems of Measurement covers the units used within each system of measurement. In addition, the student has the opportunity to practice converting units from one system of measurement to another. The module supports the following objectives:

METRIC SYSTEM

OBJECTIVES:
1. List the metric units.
2. Describe how the decimal system is used to change the value of a number.
3. Identify the metric prefixes and symbols and the numeric equivalents.
4. Identify the rules for writing metric notations.
5. Use the appropriate letters to represent the basic units of measurement.
6. Identify the beginning and the desired metric units in drug dosage calculation problems.
7. Move the decimal point to convert drug dosage problems.
8. Solve drug dosage problems using metric units.

HOUSEHOLD SYSTEM

OBJECTIVES:
1. Define the household units of measurement.
2. Write the household units of measurement using the correct abbreviations.
3. Identify equivalent measurements related to and within the household system.
4. Solve drug dosage problems using household units.

CONVERSIONS

OBJECTIVES:
1. State the metric and household equivalent measurements.
2. Use equivalent measurements or the metric line to convert the units of measurement.
3. Identify the ordered unit of measurement and the desired unit of measurement in a problem.
4. Read and interpret drug dosage calculation problems.
5. Convert the units of measurement and solve drug dosage calculation problems.

Worksheet:
Using the Metric System in Medication Administration

For extra practice, interpret the following Physician's Orders.

1.

Date	Physician's Orders
7/25	Give 0.25 g of Drug A p.o.
	Patient's name ID ********

How many mg will the nurse give? _____

2.

Date	Physician's Orders
7/25	Give 5 mg of Drug B IM.
	Patient's name ID ********

How many mcg will the nurse give? _____

3.

Date	Physician's Orders
7/25	Give 2000 mg of Drug C p.o.
	Patient's name ID ********

How many g will the nurse give? _____

4.

Date	Physician's Orders
7/25	Give 1 g of Drug D IV.
	Patient's name ID ********

How many mcg will the nurse give? _____

5.

Date	Physician's Orders
7/25	Give 20 mm of Drug E topically.
	Patient's name ID ********

How many cm will the nurse give? _____

Worksheet: Using the Household System in Medication Administration

For extra practice, interpret the following Physician's Orders.

1.

Date	Physician's Orders
7/25	**Give 2 Tbs of Drug V.**
	Patient's name ID ********

How many tsp will the nurse give? _____

Fill in the medicine cup with the ordered dose.

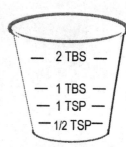

2.

Date	Physician's Orders
7/25	**Give 3 tsp of Drug W.**
	Patient's name ID ********

How many Tbs will the nurse give? _____

Fill in the medicine cup with the ordered dose.

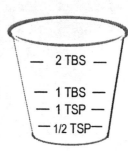

3.

Date	Physician's Orders
7/25	**Give 1 oz of Drug X.**
	Patient's name ID ********

The nurse will give _____ Tbs of Drug X.

4.

Date	Physician's Orders
7/25	**Give ½ ounce of Drug Y.**
	Patient's name ID ********

How many tsp will the nurse give? _____

Fill in the medicine cup with the ordered dose.

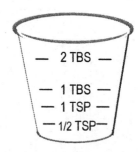

5.

Date	Physician's Orders
7/25	**Give 1 6 oz glass of juice.**
	Patient's name ID ********

How many Tbs will the nurse give? _____

Worksheet: Converting Between Systems of Measurement in Clinical Practice

For extra practice, solve the following problems:

1.

> **Convert the ordered dose and unit of measurement to the equivalent dose in milligrams.**
>
> a. ampicillin 0.5 g p.o. _____ mg   b. ampicillin 0.25 g p.o. _____ mg
> c. piperacillin 2 g IM _____ mg   d. piperacillin 3.5 g IM _____ mg
> e. levothyroxine 100 mcg p.o. _____ mg   f. levothyroxine 750 mcg p.o. _____ mg

2.

> **Convert the ordered dose and the unit of measurement to the approximate equivalent measurement.**
>
> a. milk of magnesia 15 mL p.o. _____ oz   b. milk of magnesia 30 mL p.o. _____ oz
> c. antacid A 10 mL p.o. p.r.n. _____ tsp   d. antacid A 30 mL p.o. p.r.n. _____ Tbs
> e. polyethylene glycol 2.5 L p.o. _____ mL   f. polyethylene glycol 0.4 L p.o. _____ mL

3.

> **Convert the units of measurement in the situation to the equivalent measurements in the parentheses.**
>
> a. The patient is a 35-year-old man who is 6 ft tall (_____cm) and weighs 84 kg (_____lb). He has a surgical scar 5 mm (_____cm) on the abdomen. There is a birthmark on the right leg measuring 3 inches (_____cm). He enjoys running 10 km (_____M) per day. The patient needs to be monitored for fluid loss in excess of 0.75 L (_____dL) per day.
>
> b. The MD orders $FeSO_4$ 0.3 g (_____mg) p.o. t.i.d. mixed in 2 tsp (_____mL) of applesauce, 1L (_____mL) D5W q.8h.; push oral fluids to at least 10 ounces (_____mL) q.4h. Other orders include 1/2 ounce (_____mL) of aluminum hydroxide after meals and 60 mg (g_____) of sleeping medication at night.
>
> c. On discharge, the patient is instructed to take 1 Tbs (_____mL) or (_____tsp) of aluminum hydroxide after meals, and to drink 8 glasses (_____oz) or (_____mL) and 2 cups (_____oz) or (_____mL) of herbal tea during the day.

Module: INTAKE AND OUTPUT

TO THE INSTRUCTOR:
The Intake and Output (I &O) Module presents the specifics of measuring I & O in the clinical setting. Oral and parenteral intake are covered. In addition, the module includes a section on preparation of dilute NG tube feedings.

<u>Highlights of the module</u>: Intake and Output includes practical information about measuring and calculating I & O. Clinical case studies vary from simple to complex. Content includes what is (and what is not) measured as I & O, IV intake, and calculating intake when an IV infusion has stopped or a rate change has been ordered. Practice in solving clinical I & O problems is included. The module supports the following objectives:

INTAKE AND OUTPUT

OBJECTIVES:
1. Identify the equipment used to measure oral intake.
2. Calculate oral intake.
3. Identify the equipment used to measure output.
4. Calculate output.
5. Calculate output for the patient with a bladder irrigation.

PARENTERAL INTAKE

OBJECTIVES:
1. Identify common terminology related to IV therapy.
2. Calculate parenteral intake from the primary IV.
3. Calculate parenteral intake from the IVPB.
4. Solve parenteral intake problems.

TUBE FEEDINGS

OBJECTIVES:
1. Identify important information on the label of a prepared tube feeding formula.
2. Identify the types of enteral feeding tubes.
3. Name the components of an order for enteral tube feedings.
4. Define full-strength and dilute tube feedings.
5. Solve problems that require dilution of formula tube feedings.

Worksheet:
Intake and Output

For extra practice, solve the following problems.

1. The patient was n.p.o. for breakfast but was started on a clear liquid diet for lunch. For lunch, the patient took ½ of a 6 oz cup of tea, 6 ounces of broth, and approximately 3 ounces of JELL-O®. The patient's indwelling urinary catheter was emptied at 1400, and 475 mL of yellow urine was measured. The patient had one liquid stool at 1030 measuring 200 mL, and a formed stool at 1300. Throughout the shift, the primary IV was infusing at 125 mL / hr.

Intake and Output					
	oral	IV	urine	emesis	other
7 – 3	360	1000	cath. 475	diar	rhea 200
total	360	1000	475	—	200
3 – 11					
total					
11 – 7					
total					
24-hr total					

The nurse charted the following on the patient's I & O record. Is the charting correct?

_____

2. At 1230, the nurse collects the patient's lunch tray. The lunch tray contains the following:

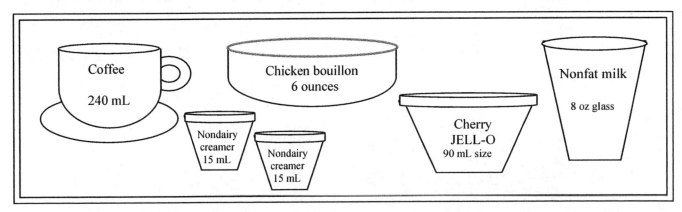

Coffee 240 mL

Nondairy creamer 15 mL

Nondairy creamer 15 mL

Chicken bouillon 6 ounces

Cherry JELL-O 90 mL size

Nonfat milk 8 oz glass

a. The patient took approximately ½ of the coffee with creamers added, all of the bouillon and JELL-O, and approximately ¼ of the milk. Calculate the patient's intake.

_____

b. If the patient had taken 100% of the tray, the patient's intake would be:

_____

3. For breakfast, the patient drank 1 cup of coffee and 3 ounces of orange juice, and ate approximately 4 ounces of Cream of Wheat® and 2 slices of toast. The patient vomited 80 mL of yellow liquid at 1030. For lunch, the patient took 1 cup of tea and 2 ounces of JELL-O. The patient voided twice during the shift (325 mL and 190 mL). The licensed vocational nurse emptied the patient's two wound drains at 1400. Drain #1 contained 50 mL of serosanguineous fluid. Drain #2 contained 7 mL of dark red fluid. The patient's IV ran at 75 mL / hr throughout the shift. Record the patient's I & O for the day shift on the I & O record below.

Intake and Output

	oral	IV	urine	emesis	other
7 – 3					
total					

4. During the 11 – 7 shift, the patient was n.p.o. except for ice chips. During the shift, he had approximately 100 mL of ice chips. The patient vomited 35 mL at 0300. The nursing assistant emptied the patient's indwelling urinary catheter at 0600, and recorded 375 mL on the I & O record. The patient had diarrhea 3 times during the night. The liquid stool measured 90 mL, 120 mL, and 60 mL. Throughout the shift, the primary IV was infusing at 150 mL / hr.

Intake and Output

	oral	IV	urine	emesis	other
7 – 3	370	1000	cath. 475		diarrhea 120
total	370	1000	475		120
3 – 11	90	1175	cath. 350	65	
total	90	1175	350	65	
11 – 7					
total					
24-hr total					

Chart the night shift intake and output on the patient's I & O record.

Then, calculate the 24-hour I & O.

I _____

O _____

5. During the 3 – 11 shift, the patient had a continuous bladder irrigation running at 100 mL / hr. At the end of the shift, the nursing assistant reported that she emptied a total of 1325 mL from the catheter bag. The nurse emptied the patient's wound drains at 2200. The first drained 30 mL and the second drained 85 mL. The NG tube drained 250 mL for the shift. What is the patient's total output for the 3 – 11 shift?

_____

Worksheet:
Parenteral Intake

For extra practice, solve the following problems.

1. The patient had a primary IV infusing at 75 mL / hr. In addition, the doctor ordered two IVPB medications: metronidazole 500 mg IVPB in 100 mL D5W q.6h. (0800 - 1400 - 2000 - 0200) and cefotaxime 1 g in 50 mL NS q.12h. (1000 - 2200).

Intake and Output					
	oral	IV	urine	emesis	other
7 – 3		600 150			
total		750			
3 – 11		600 150			
total		750			
11 – 7		600 100			
total		700			
24-hr total		2200			

Look at the patient's I & O record. Is the charting correct for the 24-hour period?

_____

2. The patient has an order for 1 L D5/0.45 NS with 20 mEq KCl q.10h. At 0700, the start of the shift, there was 700 mL of IV fluid in the IV bag. The IV infiltrated at 1130, and was restarted at 1230. What is the parenteral intake for the 0700 – 1500 shift?

_____

3. In the morning report, the day shift nurse learned that the patient's IV (D5NS at 80 mL / hr with 300 mL remaining in the bag) had infiltrated at 0630. The IV was restarted on the day shift at 0730. The nurse gave the patient an IVPB of 50 mL D5W with 500 mg ampicillin at 1000. At 12 noon, the MD increased the rate to 100 mL / hr. The patient pulled out the IV at 1230, and the nurse restarted it again at 1330. What is the patient's parenteral intake from 0700 to 1500?

_____

4. The following orders were noted by the 7 – 3 shift nurse.

5/12 1. 1 L D5/0.45 NS q.8h.(Started @ 0930.)
      2. 1 unit whole blood (500 mL) over 3 hours. (Start infusion after 1st cimetidine dose.) **(Blood started @ 1030.)**
      3. Cimetidine 300 mg IVPB in 50 mL NS over 15 min.q.6h. (Give 1st dose at 1000.). **(given @ 0945)** Signature, MD

      ———— **Noted, S. Nurse, RN 5/12 0900**

The patient has two IV sites. The primary IV runs continuously. Calculate the parenteral intake from 0700 – 1500.

_____

For extra practice, solve the following problems.

1. The doctor wrote an order for a full-strength tube feeding for a patient with a PEG tube. Twenty-four hours later the patient developed diarrhea. The nurse called the doctor and received a new order as follows:

8/21	Change PEG tube feeding to ½-strength Glucerna. Run at 40 mL / hr.
	Signature, MD

    The nurse obtained a can of Glucerna®. The tube feeding formula can contained 237 mL. How much water will the nurse add to the can of tube feeding to make a ½-strength formula?

    _____

2. The patient has an order for ¼-strength tube feedings. The following can of tube feeding formula is sent up from the kitchen. How many mL of water will the nurse add to the can to make a ¼-strength solution?

    _____

    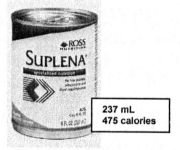

    237 mL
    475 calories

3. The order is as follows:

6/12	Insert NG tube after radiographic confirmation of placement, start NS @ 30 mL / hr for 6 hours, then begin ¾-strength tube feeding of Pulmocare. Run at 45 mL / hr.
	Signature, MD

    a. The Pulmocare® can contains 237 mLof formula. How many mL of water will the nurse need to add to make a ¾-strength tube feeding?

    _____

    b. What is the total volume of the mixed solution?

    _____

    c. If the NS is started at 1330, when will the Pulmocare tube feeding be started?

    _____

4. The physician writes an order for tube feedings on the patient with a gastric tube. The order is for full-strength Glucerna at 50 mL / hr. The pharmacy sends a ready-to-hang bag of Glucerna.

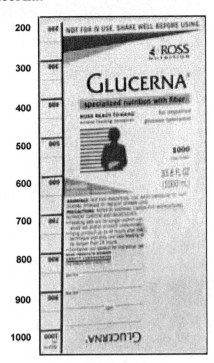

1000 cal / L

33.8 fl oz

1000 mL

a. How many mL are contained in the ready-to-hang bag of Glucerna?

_____

b. How many calories will the patient receive in 24 hours if the tube feeding formula infuses at 50 mL / hr?

_____

c. The bag of Glucerna is hung at 0200. When must a new bag of tube feeding be hung?

_____

d. The tube feeding runs at 50 mL / hr for 6 hours, then the physician increases the rate to 70 mL / hr. What is the new completion time of the tube feeding?

_____

5. The order is as follows. The nurse has the following can of Nepro®:

3/19 250 mL bolus tube feeding of 1/3-strength Nepro q.6h. (1000 - 1600 - 2200 - 0400). Follow each bolus feeding with 100 mL tap water for hydration.   Signature, MD

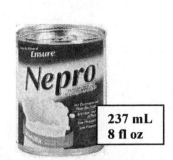

237 mL
8 fl oz

a. How much water will the nurse add to the can of Nepro to make a 1/3-strength solution?

_____

b. How many mL will the 3 – 11 shift nurse record on the I & O record for 8 hours of NG intake?

_____

Module: READING MEDICATION LABELS

TO THE INSTRUCTOR:
The Reading Medication Labels Module teaches students to identify and interpret the information found on a medication label.

<u>Highlights of the module</u>: The module uses actual medication labels to help students become acquainted with the medication label information. The dosage strength and frequently used units of measurement in medication administration are covered. The module supports the following objectives:

READING MEDICATION LABELS

OBJECTIVES:
1. Identify the essential components found on a drug label.
   - Trade name
   - Generic name
   - Form of the drug
   - Dosage strength
   - Route of administration
   - Instructions for mixing
   - Recommended dose
   - Expiration date
2. Identify the useful components found on a drug label.
   - Storage information
   - Total quantity
   - Controlled substance symbol
   - Manufacturer's name
   - Lot number

THE DOSAGE STRENGTH AND THE UNITS OF MEASUREMENT

OBJECTIVES:
1. Identify the units of measurement on drug labels.
2. List the units of measurement commonly used in nursing practice.

Worksheet:
Reading Medication Labels in Medication Administration

For extra practice, look at the drug labels and answer the corresponding questions. For all incorrect information, write the correct answer.

1.

```
        0.5 mL        1 mL      1.5 mL       2 mL
|| |||| |  |  |  |  |  |  |  |  |  |  |  |  |  |  |  |
1 mL Carpuject®      Rx only   NDC 0409-1312-30    RL-0744 (12/04)
Sterile Cartridge Unit with Luer Lock
HYDROmorphone  C II
HCl Injection, USP              (01) 0 030409 131230 2
  2 mg/mL        Warning: May be habit forming.
                 PROTECT FROM LIGHT
Hospira, Inc., Lake Forest, IL 60045 USA    Hospira
```

a. The trade name is Hydromorphone.

◎ Yes _____

◎ No _____

b. The dosage strength is 2 mg / mL .

◎ Yes _____

◎ No _____

c. The drug is a controlled subtance.

◎ Yes _____

◎ No _____

d. Storage instructions are given.

◎ Yes _____

◎ No _____

e. The total amount of drug is 2.5 mL.

◎ Yes _____

◎ No _____

2.

```
50 mL    MULTIPLE-DOSE          NDC 0409-4275-01
                            FOR INFILTRATION AND NERVE BLOCK. Not for
                            epidural and caudal use. Contains preservative.
       LIDOCAINE HCl   Each mL contains lidocaine hydrochloride,
0.5%                        anhydrous 5 mg; sodium chloride 8 mg;
       Injection, USP       methylparaben 1 mg added as preservative.
                            May contain HCl and/or NaOH for pH adjustment.
       5 mg/mL              pH 6.5 (5.0 to 7.0). Sterile, nonpyrogenic. Usual
                            dosage: See insert. Store at 20 to 25°C (68 to 77°F).
                            [See USP Controlled Room Temperature.]
HOSPIRA, INC., LAKE FOREST, IL 60045 USA   Rx only   RL-1267 (3/05)   Hospira
```

a. The trade name is Lidocaine 0.5%.

◎ Yes _____

◎ No _____

b. The dosage 5 mg / mL.

◎ Yes _____

◎ No _____

c. The drug is for single use.

◎ Yes _____

◎ No _____

d. Storage instructions are given.

◎ Yes _____

◎ No _____

e. This drug is administered IM.

◎ Yes _____

◎ No _____

3.

NDC 0172-**5311**-60

CIPROFLOXACIN
TABLETS USP

250 mg*

Rx only
100 TABLETS (White to Off-White)

IVAX Pharmaceuticals, Inc.

a. The generic name is ciprofloxacin.

◎ Yes _____

◎ No _____

b. The total quantity is 100 tablets.

◎ Yes _____

◎ No _____

c. The expiration date is necessary for the administration of the drug.

◎ Yes _____

◎ No _____

d. The dosage strength is 250 mg.

◎ Yes _____

◎ No _____

e. The route of administration is p.o.

◎ Yes _____

◎ No _____

4.

2 mL   NDC 0409-1187-01
Droperidol Inj., USP
5 mg/2 mL (2.5 mg/mL)
I.V. or I.M. Use.
Protect from light.   Rx only
RL-0634 (10/04)
Hospira, Inc.
Lake Forest, IL 60045 USA

a. The generic name is Droperidol.

◎ Yes _____

◎ No _____

b. The dosage strength is 5 mg / mL.

◎ Yes _____

◎ No _____

c. The total amount of drug is 2 mL.

◎ Yes _____

◎ No _____

d. The drug is a controlled substance.

◎ Yes _____

◎ No _____

e. The route of administration is IM or IV.

◎ Yes _____

◎ No _____

5.

100 Tablets   Rx only

INFATABS®
Dilantin® (50)
(Phenytoin Tablets, USP)

50 mg

Chewable/Flavored for Pediatric Patients
For in-institution use only
Distributed by
Pfizer **Parke-Davis**
Division of Pfizer Inc, NY, NY 10017

a. The dosage strength of the Dilantin is 50 mg / 100 tablets.

◎ Yes _____

◎ No _____

6.

10mg
NDC 0029-3210-13

PAXIL®
PAROXETINE HCl
TABLETS
1 0

30 Tablets   Scored Tablets

gsk GlaxoSmithKline   R only

a. The generic name is Paxil.

◎ Yes _____

◎ No _____

b. The total quantity is 30 tablets.

◎ Yes _____

◎ No _____

c. Storage information is provided.

◎ Yes _____

◎ No _____

d. The tablets can be divided in half evenly.

◎ Yes _____

◎ No _____

e. The route of administration is p.o.

◎ Yes _____

◎ No _____

7.

R only
See package insert for
complete product information.
Store at controlled room
temperature 20° to 25°C
(68° to 77°F) (see USP).
Each mL contains:
ibutilide fumarate, 0.1 mg;
sodium chloride, 8.90 mg;
sodium acetate trihydrate,
0.189 mg; water for injection.
When necessary, pH was
adjusted with sodium hydroxide
and/or hydrochloric acid.
Pharmacia & Upjohn Company
A subsidiary of
Pharmacia Corporation
Kalamazoo, MI 49001, USA

LOT / EXP
816416504

NDC 0009-3794-01
10 mL

Corvert®
Ibutilide fumarate
injection

1 mg/10 mL
(0.1 mg/mL)
Single-Dose Vial
For IV use only

a. The generic name is ibutilide fumarate.

◎ Yes _____

◎ No _____

b. The dosage strength is 0.1 mg / mL.

◎ Yes _____

◎ No _____

c. This is a multidose vial.

◎ Yes _____

◎ No _____

8.

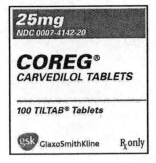

25mg
NDC 0007-4142-20

COREG®
CARVEDILOL TABLETS

100 TILTAB® Tablets

gsk GlaxoSmithKline   R only

a. The dosage strength is 25 mg.

◎ Yes _____

◎ No _____

b. The generic name is carvedilol.

◎ Yes _____

◎ No _____

Module: ORAL MEDICATIONS

TO THE INSTRUCTOR:
The Oral Medications Module introduces students to the forms of solid and liquid medications used for oral administration. The measuring equipment used to administer solid and liquid oral medications is presented. In addition, military time is taught and used throughout the module.

<u>Highlights of the module</u>: Oral Medications helps students identify the components of a medication order. Examples of physician's orders and medication administration records are used to help students see how medication orders are transcribed in the clinical setting. The students have the opportunity to evaluate transcribed orders and practice calculating oral drug dosage calculation problems. The module supports the following objectives:

INTRODUCTION TO ORAL DRUGS

OBJECTIVES:
1. Discuss the various oral drug forms.
2. Identify the oral medication routes.
3. Measure liquid drug doses using the most appropriate equipment.
4. Identify the parts of a medication order.
5. Interpret the frequency of administration of drugs.

CALCULATIONS FOR ORAL DRUGS

OBJECTIVES:
1. Define the Six Rights of Medication Administration.
2. Transcribe medication orders.
3. Use military time on the medication administration record.
4. Use the ordered amount and the dosage strength to solve drug dosage calculation problems.
5. Convert the units of measurement in drug dosage calculation problems.

For extra practice, look at the Physician's Orders and the transcribed order on the Medication Record. Ensure that the transcribed information follows the Six Rights of Medication Administation. For all incorrectly transcribed orders, write the information that would correct the problem.

1.

Date	Physician's Orders
7/29	KCl 20 mEq tab i p.o. t.i.d.
	Patient A

Date	Medication Record	
7/29	KCl 20 mEq tab i p.o. t.i.d.	0900 1300 1700
	Patient O	

☐ The medication order is transcribed correctly.

☐ The medication order is transcribed incorrectly.

_____

_____

2.

Date	Physician's Orders
7/29	Terazosin 2 mg p.o. daily at bedtime.
	Patient O

Date	Medication Record	
7/29	Terazosin 2 mg p.o. daily at bedtime.	1000
	Patient O	

☐ The medication order is transcribed correctly.

☐ The medication order is transcribed incorrectly.

_____

_____

3.

Date	Physician's Orders
7/29	Aluminum hydroxide 1 ounce p.o. p.c.
	Patient B

Date	Medication Record	
7/29	Aluminum hydroxide 1 ounce p.o. p.c.	0900 1300 1700
	Patient B	

☐ The medication order is transcribed correctly.

☐ The medication order is transcribed incorrectly.

_____

_____

4.

Date	Physician's Orders
7/29	Erythromycin oral suspension 250 mg p.o. t.i.d. q.8h.
	Patient D

Date	Medication Record	
7/29	Erythromycin oral suspension 250 mg p.o. t.i.d. q.8h.	0900 1300 1700
	Patient D	

☐ The medication order is transcribed correctly.

☐ The medication order is transcribed incorrectly.

_____

_____

5.

Date	Physician's Orders
7/29	FeSO$_4$ enteric coated tab i 325 mg p.o. c̄ meals t.i.d.
	Patient E

Date	Medication Record	
7/29	FeSO$_4$ enteric coated tab i 325 mg p.o. c̄ meals t.i.d. (crush tablet and give with meal).	0800 1200 1600
	Patient E	

☐ The medication order is transcribed correctly.

☐ The medication order is transcribed incorrectly.

_____

_____

6.

Date	Physician's Orders
7/29	Percocet tab i p.o. q.4h. p.r.n. pain.
	Patient T

Date	Medication Record
7/29	Percodan tab i p.o. q.4h. p.r.n. pain.
	Patient T

☐ The medication order is transcribed correctly.

☐ The medication order is transcribed incorrectly.

_____

_____

7.

Date	Physician's Orders
7/29	Digoxin 0.125 mg tab i p.o. daily.
	Patient Z

Date	Medication Record	
7/29	Digoxin 0.125 mg tab i p.o. daily.	0900
	Patient Z	

☐ The medication order is transcribed correctly.

☐ The medication order is transcribed incorrectly.

_____

_____

Worksheet:
Components of the Medication Order

Look at the ordered medication in the Physician's Orders. Ensure that all components of the medication order are written. For all incorrect medication orders, identify the component of the order that is missing, and check the most appropriate follow-up action.

1.

Date	Physician's Orders
8/1	Methicillin 250 mg tab i p.o.
	Patient S

☐ The medication order is correct.

☐ The medication order is incorrect.

_____

_____

Clinical action

☐ Give the medication as ordered.
☐ Call the pharmacist.
☐ Leave a note for the MD on the patient's chart to clarify the order.
☐ Call the MD.
☐ Give a dose and call the MD.

2.

Date	Physician's Orders
8/1	Allopurinol 100 mg tab i p.o. t.i.d. x 2 days then b.i.d.
	Patient C

☐ The medication order is correct.

☐ The medication order is incorrect.

_____

_____

Clinical action

☐ Call the pharmacist.
☐ Administer the medication as ordered.
☐ Call the MD.
☐ Give for 2 days and clarify the b.i.d. order.

3.

Date	Physician's Orders
8/1	Morphine sulfate 30 mg q.3h. p.r.n. pain.
	Patient X

☐ The medication order is correct.

☐ The medication order is incorrect.

_____

_____

Clinical action

☐ Call the pharmacist.
☐ Leave a note for the MD on the patient's chart to clarify the order.
☐ Call the MD.
☐ Give a dose and call the MD.

Use the Medication Record and the drug labels to solve the following problems.

1.

Date	Medication Record	
8/1	Dilantin 0.1 g p.o. q.8h.	0500
		1300
		2100
	Patient H	

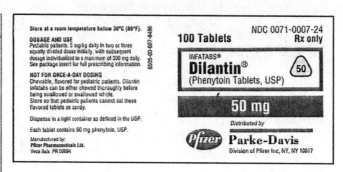

Store at a room temperature below 30°C (86°F).

DOSAGE AND USE
Pediatric patients, 5 mg/kg daily in two or three equally divided doses initially, with subsequent dosage individualized to a maximum of 300 mg daily. See package insert for full prescribing information.

NOT FOR ONCE-A-DAY DOSING
Chewable, flavored for pediatric patients. Dilantin Infatabs can be either chewed thoroughly before being swallowed or swallowed whole. Store so that pediatric patients cannot eat these flavored tablets as candy.

Dispense in a tight container as defined in the USP.

Each tablet contains 50 mg phenytoin, USP.

Manufactured by:
Pfizer Pharmaceuticals Ltd.
Vega Baja. PR 00694

NDC 0071-0007-24
100 Tablets   **Rx only**

INFATABS®
Dilantin®   ⬩50⬩
(Phenytoin Tablets, USP)

50 mg

Distributed by
Pfizer **Parke-Davis**
Division of Pfizer Inc, NY, NY 10017

For the 0500 dose, the nurse will give:

_____

2.

Date	Medication Record	
8/1	Zofran 8 mg p.o. 1 hour prior to radiation therapy treatment.	0900
	Patient D	

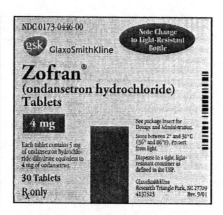

NDC 0173-0446-00

gsk GlaxoSmithKline

Note Change to Light-Resistant Bottle

Zofran®
(ondansetron hydrochloride)
Tablets

4 mg

Each tablet contains 5 mg of ondansetron hydrochloride dihydrate equivalent to 4 mg of ondansetron.

30 Tablets

R only

See package insert for Dosage and Administration. Store between 2° and 30°C (36° and 86°F). Protect from light.

Dispense in a tight, light-resistant container as defined in the USP.

GlaxoSmithKline
Research Triangle Park, NC 27709
4137523   Rev. 9/01

For the 0900 dose, the nurse will give:

_____

3.

Date	Medication Record	
8/1	Augmentin susp. 0.125 g p.o. q.12h.	0900
		2100
	Patient W	

250mg/5mL
NDC 0029-6090-23

AUGMENTIN®
AMOXICILLIN/
CLAVULANATE
POTASSIUM
FOR ORAL SUSPENSION

When reconstituted,
each 5 mL contains:
AMOXICILLIN, 250 MG,
as the trihydrate
CLAVULANIC ACID, 62.5 MG,
as clavulanate potassium

100mL
(when reconstituted)

gsk GlaxoSmithKline   R only

Shade in the desired amount in the most appropriate measuring device.

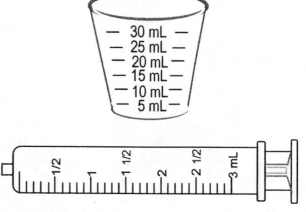

Module: SYRINGES AND NEEDLES

TO THE INSTRUCTOR:
The Syringes and Needles Module teaches the basic concepts related to reading and measuring drug dosages in syringes. Choosing the correct syringe and needle size for different medications is emphasized.

Highlights of the module: Syringes and Needles introduces the syringe, explains reading calibration lines on a syringe, and differentiates the common types of syringes used in clinical practice. The length and gauge of needles are discussed. Common syringes seen in the clinical setting are presented, and the student has an opportunity to practice drawing up doses in the syringes. The module supports the following objectives:

SYRINGES AND NEEDLES:
SYRINGES

OBJECTIVES:
1. Identify the parts of a syringe.
2. Locate the zero line on a syringe.
3. Read syringe calibrations and measure doses in a syringe.
4. Identify and read calibrations on the common syringes.
5. Choose the appropriate syringe for administration of parenteral medications.

SYRINGES AND NEEDLES:
NEEDLES

OBJECTIVES:
1. Define needle gauge.
2. Discuss the reasons for variations in needle gauge.
3. Discuss the reasons for variations in needle length.
4. Identify the needle and syringe combinations used for parenteral medication administration.
5. Choose the appropriate length and gauge of needle for parenteral injections.

Worksheet:
Using Syringes in Clinical Practice

For extra practice, solve the following problems.

1. The medication cart contains the following syringes for use in parenteral medication administration. Select the most appropriate syringe for each of the clinical situations below.

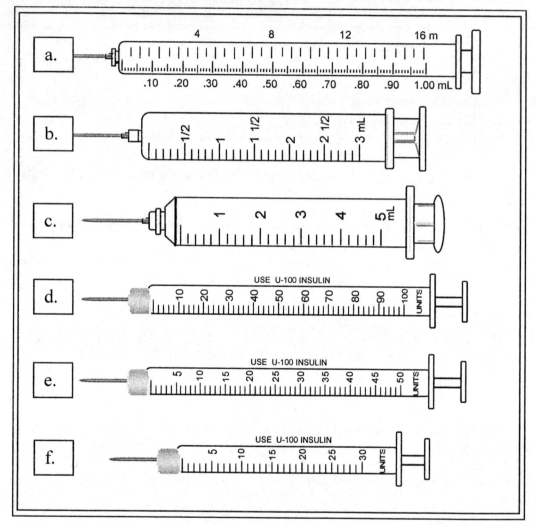

1.a. The nurse is to administer an IM injection of procaine penicillin G 600,000 units in 1 mL. Write the letter that represents the syringe needed to administer this dose.

_____

b. The nurse is to administer a subcut injection of epoetin 3000 units in 0.75 mL. Write the letter that represents the syringe needed to administer this dose.

_____

c. The nurse is to administer a subcut injection of Humulin Regular insulin 7 units and Humulin NPH insulin 12 units to a patient a.c. breakfast. Write the letter that represents the syringe needed to administer this dose.

_____

d. The nurse is to administer an ID injection of PPD 0.1 mL to a patient during an employee physical examination. Write the letter that represents the syringe needed to administer this dose.

_____

e. The nurse is to administer an IV injection of methylprednisolone 64 mg to a patient with multiple sclerosis. The ordered dose is contained in 0.8 mL. Write the letter that represents the syringe needed to administer this dose.

_____

2. Look at the medication orders below, and indicate whether the nurse has drawn up the correct amount in the syringe. If incorrect, draw a line to the correct amount.

a. Digoxin 0.58 mL IV
   Correct amount?
   _____

b. Digoxin 0.25 mL IV
   Correct amount?
   _____

c. Varicella vaccine 0.5 mL IM
   Correct amount?
   _____

d. NPH insulin 52 units subcut
   Correct amount?
   _____

e. Furosemide 4 mL IV
   Correct amount?
   _____

f. Meperidine 1.5 mL and glycopyrrolate 0.3 mL IM
   Correct amount?
   _____

g. Humulin 70/30 insulin 22 units subcut
   Correct amount?
   _____

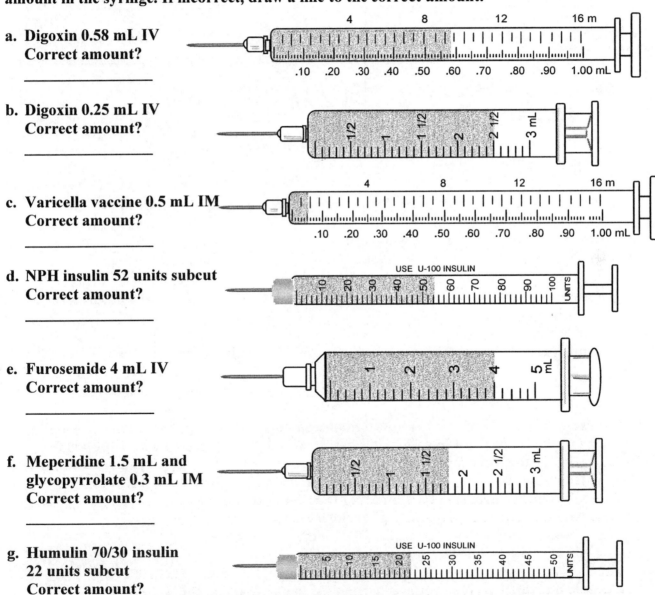

Worksheet:
Using Needles in Clinical Practice

For extra practice, solve the following problems.

The supply cart has the following needles for injection. Match the needles with the injections listed below. Fill in the box with the correct letter.

☐	26 G 3/8"	☐	18 G 1"
☐	28 G 1/2"	☐	21 G 1 1/2"
☐	25 G 5/8"	☐	22 G 2"

1. a. **Dalteparin 2500 International Units subcut on call to O.R., for a patient scheduled for total hip replacement.**

   b. **Amikacin 200 mg IM q.8h, for a 130 kg patient with a wound infection.**

   c. **Delayed-type hypersensitivity skin testing 0.1 mL of tetanus antigen ID, for a patient in the allergy clinic.**

   d. **Humulin R 4 units for blood sugar greater than 250 mg / dL, for a patient with type 2 diabetes.**

   e. **Tetanus vaccine 0.5 mL IM, for a patient with a laceration in the emergency room.**

   f. **1 mL viscous medication to be withdrawn from a vial for a stat IV push dose.**

2. **The nurse is to give a Z-track IM injection of iron dextran 100 mg. Iron dextran is highly irritating to the tissues and has the potential to cause local irritation and a brown skin discoloration at the injection site. Which of the following should the nurse do to minimize the adverse local effects of iron dextran? Discuss your thinking about the answers.**
   a. **Change the needle before injecting the iron dextran.**
   b. **Massage the site vigorously after the injection.**
   c. **Delay removing the needle for 10 seconds.**
   d. **Choose a short needle to give the injection.** _____

3. **The needle on which syringe cannot be changed to another size needle?**

   _____

Name: _____

Date: _____

Worksheet:
Syringes and Needles in Clinical Practice

For extra practice, solve the following problems.

Nurses in the clinical setting need to learn common syringe and needle sizes. Write in the standard syringe and needle size used for the following common injections:

	Syringe Volume	Needle Gauge	Needle Length
1.a. IM injection into a standard-size adult			
b. IM injection into an obese adult			
c. Subcut injection			
d. Insulin injection			
e. ID injection			
f. Withdrawing medication for IV injection			

2. The nurse reads the following orders on a patient's medication administration record:

1. **Ketorolac 60 mg IM at bedtime 9/16.**	[2200]
2. **Heparin 5000 units q.12.h. subcut**	[1000 - 2200]
3. **Morphine sulfate 5 mg IV**	
q.3 – 4h. p.r.n. severe pain (pain scale 7 – 10).	

At 2200 on 9/16, the patient is complaining of severe pain. The nurse prepares the patient's medications. Are the doses, syringes, and needles correct for administering the medications?

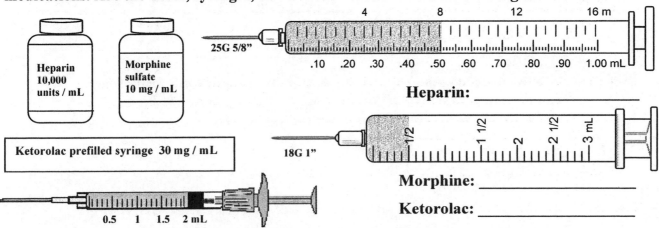

Heparin: _____

Morphine: _____

Ketorolac: _____

Module: PARENTERAL MEDICATIONS

TO THE INSTRUCTOR:
The Parenteral Medications Module assists students in learning how to use parenteral drug labels to calculate drug dosages. Students have the opportunity to practice with different units of measurement and convert units of measurement in the calculation of parenteral drug dosages.

<u>Highlights of the module:</u> Parenteral Medications covers calculation of parenteral drug dosages, including insulin, with examples using vials, ampules, prefilled syringes, and prefilled cartridges. Students can practice drawing up parenteral medication in a syringe. The module supports the following objectives:

INTRODUCTION TO PARENTERAL MEDICATIONS

OBJECTIVES:
1. Identify the parenteral routes.
2. Identify the containers used to package parenteral drugs.

THE PARENTERAL DRUG ORDER

OBJECTIVES:
1. Identify the parts of a parenteral medication order.
2. Discuss the types of parenteral orders.
3. Interpret the p.r.n. order on the medication record.

WORKING WITH INSULIN ORDERS

OBJECTIVES:
1. Identify the main types of insulin.
2. Use insulin drug labels and interpret insulin orders.
3. Interpret sliding scale insulin orders.
4. Measure the ordered amount of insulin using the appropriate insulin syringe.

CALCULATING PARENTERAL DRUG DOSAGES

OBJECTIVES:
1. Use the ordered amount and the dosage strength to solve drug dosage calculation problems.
2. Draw up the ordered amount using the appropriate syringe.

For extra practice, use the Medication Record and the drug labels to solve the following problems.

1.

Date	Medication Record
8/1	Morphine sulfate 2 mg q.3h. IV p.r.n. pain.
	Patient O

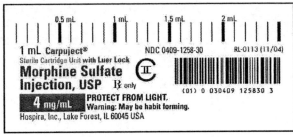

The patient complains of pain at 1200. The nurse will give:

_____

How many mL will the nurse discard from the prefilled syringe?

_____

Shade in the syringe with the amount the nurse will administer.

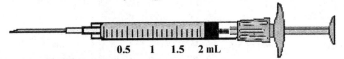

0.5   1   1.5   2 mL

2.

Date	Medication Record	
8/1	Levothyroxine 60 mcg IV daily at 0900.	0900
	Patient M	

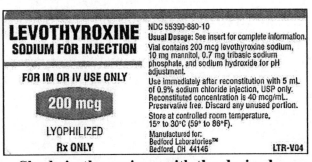

The nurse will give:

_____

Shade in the syringe with the desired amount.

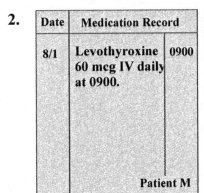

3.

Date	Medication Record
8/1	Quinidine gluconate 60 mg IM now.
	Patient H

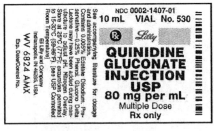

The nurse will give:

_____

Shade in the syringe with the desired amount.

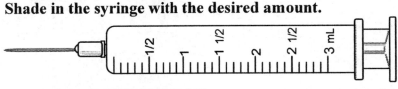

4.

Date	Medication Record	
8/2	Gentamicin 60 mg IV q.8h.	0500 1300 2100

Available:

Gentamicin
80 mg / 2 mL

Shade in the desired amount in the most appropriate syringe.

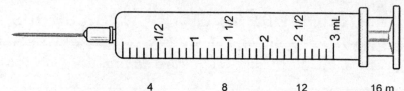

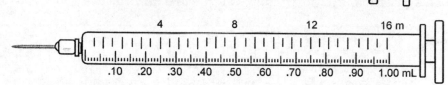

5.

Date	Medication Record	
8/1	Hydroxyzine 50 mg q.6h. IM p.r.n. anxiety.	

Available:

Hydroxyzine
100 mg / 2 mL

Shade in the desired amount in the most appropriate syringe.

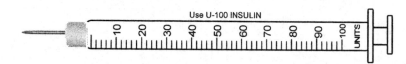

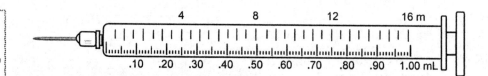

6.

Date	Medication Record	
8/1	Phytonadione 2.5 mg subcut now and repeat at 2100.	

Available:

Phytonadione
10 mg / mL

Shade in the desired amount in the most appropriate syringe.

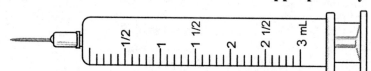

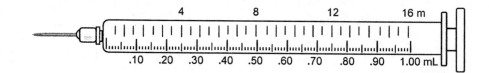

7.

Date	Medication Record	
8/1	Bumetanide 1 mg b.i.d. IV.	1000 2200

Available:

Bumetanide
0.25 mg / mL

Shade in the desired amount in the most appropriate syringe.

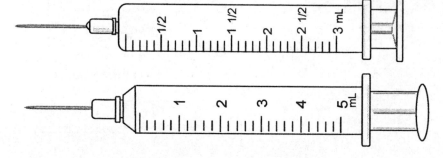

Worksheet:
Working with Insulin Orders

Use the Physician's Orders to administer the desired insulin dose for the following problems.

1.

Date	Physician's Orders
8/2	**Humulin 70/30 13 units subcut q.AM.**

Shade in the desired amount in the most appropriate syringe.

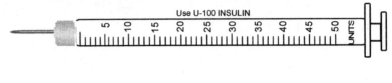
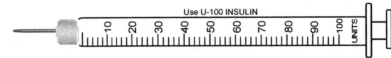

2.

Date	Physician's Orders
8/2	**Humulin N 25 units with Humulin R 7 units q.AM.**

Shade in the desired amount in the most appropriate syringe.

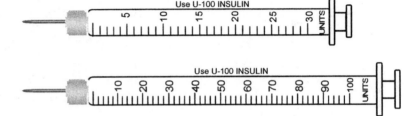

3.

Date	Physician's Orders
8/2	**Insulin orders (use regular insulin):** **If BS:** **150 – 160 give 2 units** **161 – 175 give 4 units** **176 – 200 give 6 units**

Shade in the desired amount in the most appropriate syringe.

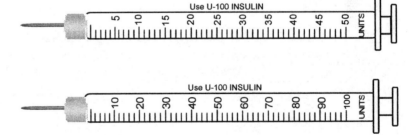

The BS is 159 mg / dL.

4.

Date	Physician's Orders
8/2	**If BS:** **150 – 175 give 3 units regular insulin** **176 – 195 give 6 units regular insulin** **196 or over, call MD**

Shade in the desired amount in the most appropriate syringe.

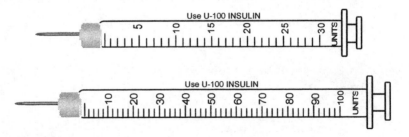

The BS is 175 mg / dL.

Module: RECONSTITUTION OF POWDERED MEDICATIONS

TO THE INSTRUCTOR:
The Reconstitution of Powdered Medications Module teaches the basic concepts relevant to mixing powdered medications and calculating the dosages of the mixed medication. Single-strength and multiple-strength reconstitution problems are discussed.

<u>Highlights of the module:</u> Reconstitution of Powdered Medications discusses the steps of reconstitution, explains reading reconstitution instructions on drug labels, and shows calculations involving reconstituted medications. Using the dosage strength in calculating dosages is stressed. The module supports the following objectives:

RECONSTITUTION OF POWDERED MEDICATIONS

OBJECTIVES:
1. Define the concept of reconstitution.
2. Determine the dosage strength obtained after reconstituting powdered drugs.
3. Write the necessary information on the medication label after reconstitution.

RECONSTITUTION OF POWDERED MEDICATIONS: SINGLE-STRENGTH RECONSTITUTION

OBJECTIVES:
1. Determine the amount and type of diluent, and the resulting dosage strength, for single-strength reconstitution problems.
2. Calculate doses of single-strength reconstituted medications.

RECONSTITUTION OF POWDERED MEDICATIONS: MULTIPLE-STRENGTH RECONSTITUTION

OBJECTIVES:
1. Determine the amount of diluent and the dosage strength obtained when mixing a powdered drug with multiple directions for reconstitution.
2. Correctly mark the medication label after reconstitution.
3. Solve multiple-strength reconstitution problems.

Worksheet: Single-Strength Reconstitution

For extra practice, solve the following problems.

1. The nurse transcribes a new order on an adult patient with bronchitis.

> 4/12 1. **Start Augmentin oral suspension 450 mg q.8h.**   Signature MD
> —————— Noted, S. Nurse, RN 4/12 1230

The nurse receives the following vial of powdered medication from the pharmacy:

Directions for mixing:
Tap bottle until all powder flows freely. Add approximately 2/3 of total water for reconstitution (total=87 mL); shake vigorously to wet powder. Add remaining water; again shake vigorously.
Dosage: See accompanying prescribing information.

Keep tightly closed.
Shake well before using.
Must be refrigerated.
Discard after 10 days.

250mg/5mL
NDC 0029-6090-23

AUGMENTIN®
AMOXICILLIN/
CLAVULANATE
POTASSIUM
FOR ORAL SUSPENSION
When reconstituted,
each 5 mL contains:
AMOXICILLIN, 250 MG,
as the trihydrate
CLAVULANIC ACID, 62.5 MG,
as clavulanate potassium

100mL
(when reconstituted)

gsk GlaxoSmithKline   R only

a. What type of diluent will the nurse add to the Augmentin® powder?   _____

b. What amount of diluent will the nurse add?   _____

c. Dosage strength of the mixed medication: _____

d. What does the number "100 mL" on the drug label represent?   _____

e. How many mL will the nurse give to the patient?   _____

f. The Augmentin powder is mixed at 1:30 PM on 4/12 and stored in the refrigerator. When will it lose its potency?

_____

2. The medication on the right has been reconstituted by the nurse on 2/24 at 10:00 PM.

Fill in the label with the information needed after reconstituting the drug.

_____

_____

_____

3. The following order is written on the patient's medication record:

7/22 Levothyroxine 100 mcg IV daily.	[2100]

The following vial is in the patient's drawer in the medication cart:

LEVOTHYROXINE SODIUM FOR INJECTION

FOR IM OR IV USE ONLY

200 mcg

LYOPHILIZED

Rx ONLY

NDC 55390-880-10
Usual Dosage: See insert for complete information.
Vial contains 200 mcg levothyroxine sodium, 10 mg mannitol, 0.7 mg tribasic sodium phosphate, and sodium hydroxide for pH adjustment.
Use immediately after reconstitution with 5 mL of 0.9% sodium chloride injection, USP only. Reconstituted concentration is 40 mcg/mL. Preservative free. Discard any unused portion.
Store at controlled room temperature, 15° to 30°C (59° to 86°F).
Manufactured for:
Bedford Laboratories™
Bedford, OH 44146   LTR-V04

a. What type of diluent will the nurse add to the levothyroxine powder? _____

b. What amount of diluent will the nurse add? _____

c. What is the dosage strength of the mixed medication? _____

d. How much will the nurse give to the patient? _____

e. Fill in the label with the information needed after reconstituting the medication.

4. The package insert of an antibiotic drug states the following:

> **ANTIBIOTIC B**
> For IM use, reconstitute with 2.5 mL Sterile Water for Injection. Shake vigorously. Provides an approximate volume of 2.8 mL. When mixed, each 0.5 mL contains 1.5 g of Antibiotic B.
> For IV use, reconstitute with 5 mL Sterile Water for Injection or Normal Saline for Injection. Shake vigorously. Provides an approximate volume of 5.5 mL. When mixed, each 1 mL contains 1.5 g of Antibiotic B.
> Store under refrigeration. Unused portion of drug stable for 48 hours after mixing.

The nurse must give 1200 mg of Antibiotic B IM.

a. What is the dosage strength once the medication is mixed? _____

b. How many mL will the nurse give to the patient? _____

c. The nurse reconstitutes the medication at 0800 on 4/17. The medication is stored in the refrigerator. On 4/19, the nurse is preparing to give a dose of Antiobiotic B at 0830. Can the dose be given from the vial that was mixed on 4/17? _____

Worksheet: Multiple-Strength Reconstitution

For extra practice, solve the following problems.

1. The patient has an order for nafcillin sodium 750 mg IV q.6h. The pharmacy sends a vial of nafcillin powder with the following instructions:

Nafcillin Sodium 1 g	
Add Sterile Water for Injection or 0.9% NaCl.	
Diluent Added (mL)	Solution Concentration
100	1 g / 100 mL
50	1 g / 50 mL
20	1 g / 20 mL

   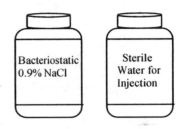

   Bacteriostatic 0.9% NaCl   Sterile Water for Injection

   a. Circle the correct vial of diluent. Choose the amount of diluent: _____

   b. How many mL of nafcillin sodium will the patient receive?   _____

   c. Fill in the nafcillin label with the appropriate information after reconstitution.

2. The patient has an order for penicillin G potassium 1 million units IV q.6h. The pharmacy sends the following vial:

   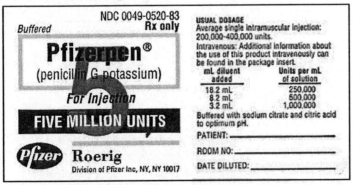

   a. Choose the amount of diluent: _____

   b. What is the dosage strength of the mixed medication?   _____

   c. How much will be given to the patient?   _____

   d. What do the five million units on the label represent?   _____

3. On 8/15, the nurse prepares to give 2:00 AM medications to the patient. The following is the medication administration record:

> 8/14 Penicillin 600,000 units IV q.8h. [1000 - 1800 - 0200]

The nurse finds the following vial of penicillin in the patient's medication drawer. The nurse on the previous shift reconstituted the medication, and labeled the vial.

> ### Penicillin Powder for Reconstitution 2 Million Units
> Diluent – Bacteriostatic Water for Injection or Normal Saline.
>
> | | units / mL of |
> |---|---|
> | Diluent Added | Mixed Medication |
> | 5   mL | 250,000 units / mL |
> | 3.5 mL | 500,000 units / mL |
> | 2 mL | 1,000,000 units / mL |
>
> 8/14
> 0930
> XX R.N.
>
> Mixed solution may be stored at room temperature for 72 hours. See accompanying package insert.
>
> Lot # xxxxxxxx   Exp. 8/XX

The nurse prepares the medication for the patient.

a. How many mL of penicillin will the patient receive? _____

b. How many doses of the medication remain in the vial after the 0200 dose on 8/15 is given? _____

c. What is the significance of the "Exp. 8/XX" at the bottom of the label on the vial? _____

4. The patient has an order for IV cefuroxime 750 mg q.12h. The pharmacy sends an ADD-Vantage® vial with a 50 mL bag of D5W. (With an ADD-Vantage system, the vial of powder is permanently attached to the IV bag and is activated by the nurse immediately before using.)

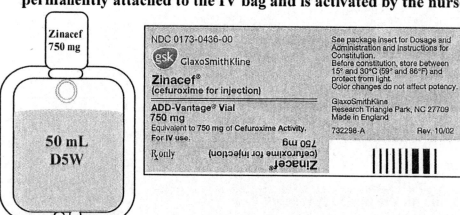

a. Check the label. Is the patient receiving the correct drug and dosage?

_____

b. The IV is to infuse over 30 minutes. What time will the IVPB be finished if the nurse starts the infusion at 1350?

_____

Module: IV CALCULATIONS

TO THE INSTRUCTOR:
The IV Calculations Module assists students in learning how to calculate mL / hr, flow rate (gtt / min), and infusion and completion time of IV fluids. The students use IV calculations in realistic clinical scenarios.

<u>Highlights of the module:</u> IV Calculations introduces students to the different sizes of IV bags and the use of the flowmeter in labeling IV bags. In addition, students obtain practice reading directions for IV push medications and calculating the rate of administration for commonly used drugs. The module supports the following objectives:

IV CALCULATIONS

OBJECTIVES:
1. Define the terms primary and secondary IV, IVPB, and IVR.
2. Describe the parts of an IV tubing.
3. Discuss IV infusion by gravity and IV infusion pump.
4. Identify the components of an order for primary IV solutions.
5. Determine the mL / hr for an IV infusing by pump.
6. Determine the flow rate of an IV infusing by gravity.

IV PUSH MEDICATIONS

OBJECTIVES:
1. Identify the information needed to safely administer a drug by the IV push route.
2. Calculate the safe rate of administration for IV push drugs.

INFUSION AND COMPLETION TIME

OBJECTIVES:
1. Identify the infusion time of IV fluid (in hours and minutes).
2. Solve IV infusion time problems.
3. Identify the completion time of IV infusions.
4. Solve IV completion time problems.

LABELING IV BAGS

OBJECTIVES:
1. Read the calibrated line markings on a flowmeter.
2. Apply a flowmeter to an IV bag.
3. Calculate the amount of IV fluid infused from the flowmeter.
4. Calculate the end time on the flowmeter.

Worksheet:
Calculating mL / hr and Flow Rate (gtt / min)

For extra practice, solve the following problems. Round mL / hr and flow rate (gtt / min) problems to the nearest whole number.

1.a. The physician orders 1000 mL Lactated Ringer's to infuse over 24 hours.
How many mL will the patient receive per hour?   _____

b. The nurse uses an IV tubing with a drop factor of 15 gtt / mL.
What are the gtt / min?   _____

2.a. The physician orders 500 mL D5W to infuse q.8h.
How many mL will the patient receive per hour?   _____

b. The nurse uses a microgtt IV tubing.
What are the gtt / min?   _____

3.a. The physician orders a primary IV of 1000 mL NS q.6h.
How many mL will the patient receive per hour?   _____

b. The nurse uses an IV tubing with a drop factor of 15 gtt / mL.
What is the flow rate?   _____

4.a. The physician orders 1 unit (270 mL) of PRBCs to infuse 1.5 hours.
How many mL will the patient receive per hour?   _____

b. The nurse uses a blood tubing labeled 10 gtt / mL.
What is the flow rate?   _____

5.a. The patient is to receive an IVPB of KCl 10 mEq in 100 mL of NS
over 60 minutes. How many mL will the patient receive per hour?   _____

b. The nurse uses an IV tubing with a drop factor of 60 gtt / mL.
What are the gtt / min?   _____

6.a. The patient is to receive an IVPB of vancomycin 0.5 g in 250 mL D5W
to infuse in 2 hours. How many mL will the patient receive per hour?   _____

b. The nurse uses an IV tubing with a drop factor of 15 gtt / mL.
What is the flow rate?   _____

Worksheet:
Calculating Infusion and Completion Times

Use military time in calculating the completion time of the following IV flow problems.

1. The doctor orders 1 L NS to infuse over 8 hours. The nurse starts the IV at 1400. At 1900, the patient pulls out the IV. The nurse restarts the IV at 2200, at the same rate. Starting with the amount of IV fluid left at 1900, calculate the <u>new</u> infusion time and the completion time of the IV.

    Infusion time_____

    Completion time_____

2. The doctor orders 1 L Lactated Ringer's to infuse at 80 mL / hr. The nurse starts the IV at 2330. At 0330, the IV infiltrates. The nurse restarts the IV at 0400, at the same rate. Starting with the amount of IV fluid left at 0300, calculate the <u>new</u> infusion time and the completion time of the IV.

    Infusion time_____

    Completion time_____

3. The doctor orders 1 L D5W to infuse at 150 mL / hr. The nurse starts the IV at 0900. At 1100, the doctor decreases the rate to 100 mL / hr. Starting with the amount of IV fluid left at 1100, calculate the <u>new</u> infusion time and the completion time of the IV.

    Infusion time_____

    Completion time_____

4. The doctor orders 500 mL NS to infuse at 50 mL / hr. The nurse starts the IV at 1200. At 1600, the doctor increases the IV rate to 100 mL / hr. Starting with the amount of IV fluid left at 1600, calculate the <u>new</u> infusion time and the completion time of the IV.

    Infusion time_____

    Completion time_____

5. The doctor orders 1000 mL D10W to infuse at 100 mL / hr. The nurse starts the IV at 2030. At 2200, the IV rate is increased to 125 mL / hr per doctor's orders. Starting with the amount of IV fluid left at 2200, calculate the <u>new</u> infusion time and the completion time of the IV.

    Infusion time_____

    Completion time_____

Name: _____

Worksheet:
Labeling IV Bags

Date: _____

1. The IV is started at 1400 and is infusing at 50 mL / hr. Label the flowmeter q.2h. Shade in the amount of IV fluid in the bag at 2000.

2. The IV is started at 0930 and is infusing at 75 mL / hr. Label the flowmeter q.2h. Shade in the amount of IV fluid in the bag at 1230.

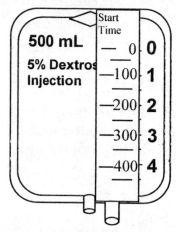

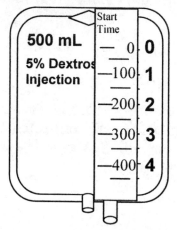

3. The IV is started at 0230 and is infusing at 125 mL / hr. Label the flowmeter hourly. Shade in the amount of IV fluid in the bag at 0630.

4. The IV is started at 2030 and is infusing at 150 mL / hr. Label the flowmeter hourly. Shade in the amount of IV fluid in the bag at 2330.

1. The PM shift nurse calculates IV intake on the patient at 2300. During the previous 8 hours, the IV has been infusing at 150 mL / hr. The nurse will take credit for how many mL of IV fluid at 2300?

_____

2. At 2330, the nurse starts a primary IV of 1 liter D5/0.45 NS, at 100 mL per hour on a newly admitted patient. The IV infiltrates at 0300, and is restarted at 0400. At 0700, the nurse calculates parenteral intake on the patient for the night shift. How many mL from the primary IV will the nurse take credit for on the night shift (2300 to 0700)?

_____

In the change of shift report at 0700, the night nurse gives credit for the number of mL remaining in the patient's IV. The amount of credit the night shift nurse will give to the day shift nurse is:

_____

3. The day shift nurse is told in the 0700 report that the patient's IV is to infuse at 50 mL / hr, and that 725 mL remain in the IV bag. How much IV credit will the day shift nurse give to the PM nurse at 1500?

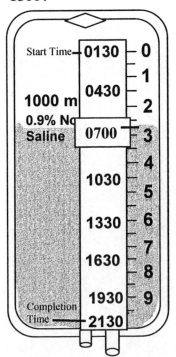

IV credit given to the PM shift at 1500:

_____

Draw a line to show the level of the IV fluid at 1500.

4. The IV is started at 2100 per MD order. Fill in the label q.2h, then write the amount of IV credit the nurse will take for the PM shift at 2300. Write the amount of IV credit the PM nurse will give to the night shift nurse at 2300.

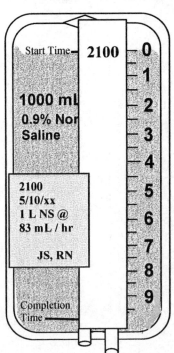

IV credit taken by the PM shift nurse at 2300:

_____

IV credit given to the night shift nurse at 2300:

_____

Draw a line to show the level of the IV fluid at 2300.

Worksheet:
IV Push Rate of Administration

1.

Date	Medication Record	
8/2	Verapamil 5 mg IVP now.	
	Patient ID BD 8-09-1932	

Drug reference information:

verapamil
(ver-ap-́a-mil)

IMPLEMENTATION
- Direct IV: Administer IV undiluted through Y-site over 2 minutes for each single dose. Administer over 3 minutes in geriatric patients.

The rate of administration for the ordered dose is:

_____

2.

Date	Medication Record	
8/2	Doxorubicin HCl 10 mg IVP now.	
	Patient ID	

Drug reference information:

High Alert

doxorubicin hydrochloride
(dox-oh-**roo**-bi-sin hye-droe-**klor**-ide)

IMPLEMENTATION
- *Rate:* Administer each dose over 3 – 5 minutes through Y-site of a free-flowing IV infusion of 0.9% NaCl or D5W. Facial flushing and erythema along involved vein frequently occur when administration is too rapid.

The rate of administration for the ordered dose is:

_____

3.

Date	Medication Record	
8/2	Atropine 1 mg IVP now.	
	Patient ID	

Drug reference information:

atropine
(at-ro-peen)

IMPLEMENTATION
- *Rate:* Administer at a rate of 0.6 mg over 1 minute. Do not add to IV solution. Inject through Y-tubing or 3-way stopcock.

The rate of administration for the ordered dose is:

_____

Module: PEDIATRIC CALCULATIONS

TO THE INSTRUCTOR:
The Pediatric Calculations Module teaches the basic concepts and practical issues involved in dosage calculation and medication administration for children. Determination of safe dose by weight and body surface area, and IV replacement of excessive fluid loss are also covered.

<u>Highlights of the module:</u> Pediatric Calculations introduces the student to variations in calculations, drug dosages, and equipment used to administer medications to children. Amounts used for parenteral injection, needle sizes, and pediatric IV equipment are discussed. Calculations related to nasogastric (NG) fluid replacement are presented. The module supports the following objectives:

PEDIATRIC CALCULATIONS

OBJECTIVES:
1. Identify two reasons why pediatric doses are different from adult doses.
2. Describe specific guidelines for oral and parenteral medication administration in children.
3. Discuss special equipment used to administer pediatric oral medications.
4. Discuss special equipment used to administer pediatric parenteral medications.

DETERMINING SAFE DOSE:
DOSAGE BASED ON BODY WEIGHT

OBJECTIVES:
1. Identify pertinent information regarding recommended dosages in the drug literature.
2. Calculate safe medication doses based on a child's body weight.

DETERMINING SAFE DOSE:
DOSAGE BASED ON BODY SURFACE AREA

OBJECTIVES:
1. Determine body surface area using the West nomogram.
2. Determine body surface area using a formula.
3. Calculate safe doses of medication based on a child's body surface area.

NASOGASTRIC FLUID REPLACEMENT

OBJECTIVES:
1. Discuss the purpose of NG fluid replacement.
2. Identify the components of an order for NG fluid replacement.
3. Identify the information needed to solve fluid replacement problems.
4. Calculate the rate of administration, infusion time, and completion time of the replacement IV fluid.

Worksheet:
Administering Medications to Children

For extra practice, solve the following problems.

1. The medication administration record for a 7-year-old hospitalized child who has been exposed to meningitis has the following medications listed:

Amoxicillin 250 mg p.o. t.i.d.	[1000 - 1800 - 0200]
Rifampin 150 mg p.o. b.i.d.	[1000 - 2200]
Multivitamin i daily	[1000]
Acetaminophen 320 mg q.4h. p.r.n. pain, or temperature greater than 101.	

    At 0945, the nursing assistant tells the nurse that the patient's vital signs are 100.1–114–28–98/56. The patient is complaining that his head hurts. The medication record states that the patient had acetaminophen 320 mg at 0530 for pain. The nurse finds the following medications in the medication drawer. Circle the medications that the nurse will give to the child at 1000.

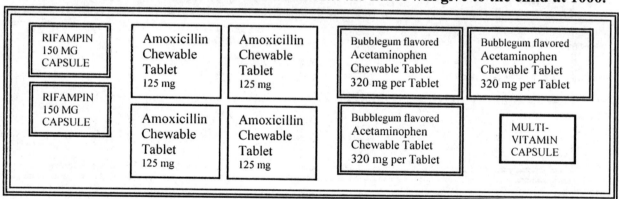

2. The medication administration record for a 2-year-old child with tetralogy of Fallot lists the following medications:

Digoxin 0.15 mg p.o. daily	[2200]
KCl 10 mEq p.o. b.i.d.	[1000 - 2200]
Furosemide 20 mg p.o. daily	[1000]

    The nurse needs to decide how best to adminster the medications to the child. Circle the best choice for each medication below.

    <u>Digoxin</u>
    a. Elixir: 0.05 mg / mL in oral syringe
    b. Tablets: 0.25 mg in med cup

    <u>Furosemide</u>
    a. Tablets: 20 mg in med cup
    b. Oral solution: 10 mg / mL in med cup

    <u>KCl</u>
    a. Chewable tablets: 10 mEq in med cup
    b. Oral solution: 30 mEq in 15 mL in med spoon

Worksheet:
Determining Safe Dose

For extra practice, solve the following problems.

1. The medication administration record for a 5-year-old child with acute lymphocytic leukemia has the following medications listed:

Vincristine 1.2 mg IV Tuesdays	[1100]
Asparaginase 18,000 International Units daily IV. Start 9/23.	[1000]
Prednisone 15 mg p.o. q.i.d.	[0800 - 1200 - 1800 - 2200]

    The child weighs 44 lb and has a BSA of 0.74 m^2. The nurse looks up the dosage information in the drug reference book. Use the information below to determine whether the ordered doses of medication are safe doses.

High Alert	High Alert	
vincristine **ROUTE AND DOSAGE** **IV (Children weighing more than 10 kg):** 1.5 – 2 mg / m^2 single dose; may repeat weekly. **IV (Children less than 10 kg):** 50 mcg / kg single dose; may repeat weekly.	**asparaginase** **ROUTE AND DOSAGE** Multiple-Agent Induction Regimen (in combination with vincristine and prednisone) **IV (Children):** 1000 International Units / kg / day for 10 successive days beginning on day 22 of regimen.	**prednisone** **ROUTE AND DOSAGE** PO (Children): 0.05 – 2 mg / kg p.o. daily in divided doses q.i.d.

    Vincristine: Maximum safe dose: _____   Is ordered dose safe? _____

    Asparaginase: Maximum safe dose: _____   Is ordered dose safe? _____

    Prednisone: Maximum safe dose: _____   Is ordered dose safe? _____

2. The medication administration record for a 10-year-old child who weighs 88 lb lists the following medications:

Cefuroxime 750 mg IV q.12h.	[1000 - 2200]
Amikacin 200 mg IV q.8h.	[0800 - 1600 - 0000]

    Use the information below to determine if the ordered doses of medication are safe doses.

Cefuroxime **ROUTE AND DOSAGE** IM, IV (Children older than 3 mo): 16.7 – 33.3 mg / kg q.8h., *or* 15 – 50 mg / kg q.12h.	**Amikacin** **ROUTE AND DOSAGE** IM, IV (Adults and Children and older infants): 5 mg / kg q.8h., or 7.5 mg / kg q.12h.

    Cefuroxime: Maximum safe dose: _____   Is ordered dose safe? _____

    Amikacin: Maximum safe dose: _____   Is ordered dose safe? _____

Worksheet:
Nasogastric Fluid Replacement

For extra practice, solve the following problems.

1. The nurse transcribes the following physician's orders for an 8-year-old child:

2/16 1. N.P.O.
2. Insert NG tube to low continuous suction.
3. IV D5/0.225 NS with 10 mEq KCl per 500 mL @ 60 mL / hr.
4. q.4h. measure and replace NG output mL for mL with 2nd IV of D5/0.45 NS with 10 mEq per 500 mL.
5. Patient to receive no more than 85 mL / hr IV intake.
— Noted, S. Nurse, RN 2/16 0930

Four hours after the NG is inserted, the nurse measures 68 mL of dark green drainage from the child's NG tube. The nurse starts the replacement IV at 1400.

a. What is the maximum rate for the replacement IV? _____

b. What is the infusion time for the replacement IV? _____

c. If the replacement IV is started at 1430, when will it be completed? _____

2. The nurse reads the following orders on a 13-year-old child's care plan:

GI System	**IV Fluids**
1. N.P.O.	1. IV: 1 L D5/0.33 NS @ 100 mL / hr.
2. NG tube to low continuous suction.	2. Replace NG output mL for mL with 2nd IV of D5/0.45 NS with 10 mEq KCl per 500 mL.
3. Measure and chart NG output q.8h.	3. Maximum hourly IV intake: 140 mL / hr.

At 1600, the nurse measures 138 mL of NG drainage. The nurse starts the replacement IV with D5/0.45 NS with 10 mEq KCl per 500 mL at 1615.

a. What is the maximum rate for the replacement IV? _____

b. What is the infusion time for the replacement IV? _____

c. When will the replacement IV be completed? _____

Module: TITRATION OF IV MEDICATIONS

TO THE INSTRUCTOR:
The Titration of IV Medications Module teaches the student about titration and the calculations needed to solve titration problems. Common and critical care IV medications are included, and the student has a choice of method for solving the problems.

<u>Highlights of the module:</u> Titration of IV Medications introduces the student to the concept of titrated medications and the use of titration in clinical practice. Titration problems frequently seen on the clinical unit are introduced. In addition, complex titration problems seen most often in the critical care area are covered. The module supports the following objectives:

INTRODUCTION TO TITRATION

OBJECTIVES:
1. Define the concept of titration.
2. Differentiate titration problems from other IV problems.
3. List the information needed to set up a titration problem.
4. Select important information from a titration problem.

SOLVING COMMON TITRATION PROBLEMS

OBJECTIVES:
1. Identify the information needed to set up a titration problem.
2. Correctly set up common titration problems.
3. Solve common titration problems.

SOLVING ADVANCED TITRATION PROBLEMS

OBJECTIVES:
1. Recognize variations in titration problems.
2. Solve a variety of advanced titration problems, including those with dosage ranges, and those with doses ordered per minute.

For extra practice, solve the following problems.

1. The order sheet for the patient includes the following order:

The pharmacy sends the following IV:

Date	Physician's Orders
3/18	**Start IV heparin infusion @ 700 units / hr.** Signature, MD Patient's name ID ********

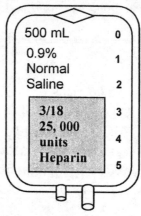

How many mL will the nurse set on the IV pump to deliver the ordered dose?

_____

2. The patient has an order for morphine sulfate 2 mg / hr via infusion pump. The IV sent from the pharmacy is labeled 100 mg morphine in 500 mL D5W. How many mL / hr will the patient receive?

_____

3. In the shift report on the cardiac unit, the nurse is told that the patient has an IV of 500 mL NS, with 125 mg diltiazem HCl infusing at 32 mL / hr via infusion pump. How many mg / hr of diltiazem are infusing?

_____

4. The patient has an IV drip of hydromorphone infusing at 15 mL / hr via an infusion pump. The order is for a continuous IV infusion of hydromorphone at 1.5 mg / hr. The IV contains 50 mg of hydromorphone in 500 mL NS. Is the patient receiving the correct dose of IV hydromorphone?

_____

5. The patient is to receive a continuous IV infusion of aminocaproic acid. The ordered dose is 1.2 g / hr. The pharmacy sends an IV of 250 mL D5NS with 15 g of amincaproic acid. How many mL / hr will the nurse set on the IV pump?

_____

6.a. The patient is to receive an IV drip of regular insulin at 6 units / hr. The pharmacy has added 50 units of the following insulin to a bag of 500 mL 0.45/NS. How many mL / hr should the patient receive?

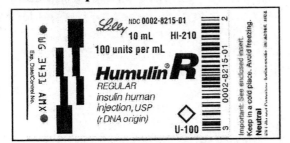

_____

b. The physician increases the insulin dosage to 8 units / hr. How many mL / hr will the nurse set on the IV pump?

_____

7. The order sheet for the patient includes the following order:

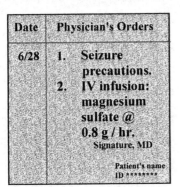

Date	Physician's Orders
6/28	1. Seizure precautions. 2. IV infusion: magnesium sulfate @ 0.8 g / hr. Signature, MD Patient's name ID ********

The pharmacy sends the following IV:

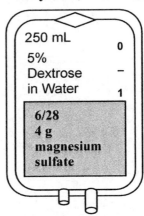

250 mL
5% Dextrose in Water

0
–
1

6/28
4 g magnesium sulfate

How many mL will the nurse set on the IV pump to deliver the ordered dose?

_____

8. The patient is to receive an IV infusion of heparin sodium at 900 units / hr. The pharmacy sends an IV of 250 mL NS with 25,000 units of heparin sodium. How many mL / hr will the nurse set on the IV pump?

_____

Worksheet:
Complex Titration Problems in Critical Care

For extra practice, solve the following problems.

1. The medication administration record for a patient in the critical care unit has the following medications listed:

    IV dobutamine 5 – 10 mcg / kg / min. Titrate to keep diastolic BP greater than 60.

    IV lidocaine 1 – 4 mg / min. Titrate for multifocal premature ventricular contractions.

    The patient weighs 55 kg. On initial assessment, the nurse finds the following IV infusions running:

    #1

    | 250 mL |
    | 5% |
    | Dextrose |
    | in Water |

    0
    –
    1

    7/20
    250 mg
    dobutamine
    added.

    #2

    | 250 mL |
    | 5% |
    | Dextrose |
    | in Water |

    0
    –
    1

    7/20
    1 g
    lidocaine
    added.

    IV #1 is infusing at 10 mL / hr per IV pump.

    IV #2 is infusing at 15 mL / hr per IV pump.

    a. What is the ordered dosage range for dobutamine in mg / hr?

    _____

    b. Is the infusion rate of dobutamine on the infusion pump set correctly?

    _____

    c. What is the ordered dosage range for lidocaine in mg / hr?

    _____

    d. Is the infusion rate of lidocaine on the infusion pump set correctly?

    _____

2.a. A patient with chest pain has an IV infusion of nitroglycerin. The physician's orders are to "infuse the nitroglycerin at a rate of 10 – 30 mcg / minute. Titrate to effect". The pharmacy sent a premixed IV of 100 mg nitroglycerin in 500 mL D5W. What rate will the nurse set on the IV infusion pump to deliver the minimum amount of nitroglycerin / hr?

_____

  b. What rate will the nurse set on the IV infusion pump to deliver the maximum amount of nitroglycerin / hr?

_____

3. The nurse transcribes the following physician's orders for a critical care patient who weighs 176 lb:

> 4/8   1. Milrinone lactate 20 mg in 150 mL D5W.
>   Infuse at a rate of 1.3 – 3 mcg / kg / min.
>   Noted, S. Nurse, RN 4/8 0930

3.a. What is the minimum rate / hr for the milrinone lactate infusion?

_____

  b. What is the maximum rate / hr for the milrinone lactate infusion?

_____

4. The order is for amiodarone 1 mg / minute per IV infusion. The pharmacy sends an IV of 360 mg amiodarone in 250 mL D5W. How many mL / hr will the nurse set on the IV pump?

_____

5. The order is for aminophylline 0.5 mg / kg / hr for a patient who weighs 50 kg. The pharmacy sends an IV of 50 mg of aminophylline in 250 mL D5W. How many mL / hr will the nurse set on the IV pump?

_____

Module: PREPARATION FOR NCLEX

TO THE INSTRUCTOR:

This section of the program presents problems similar to those found in the National Council Licensure Examination (NCLEX), and can be used to supplement the student's practice and preparation for drug dosage problems on this exam (NCLEX-RN or NCLEX-PN).

The National Council of State Boards of Nursing Testing Service currently includes test items in a variety of formats. These include:

- standard, four-option, multiple-choice items,
- multiple-choice items that require more than one response,
- fill-in-the-blank items in which a candidate must type in a numerical answer for a calculation question,
- items asking a candidate to identify an area on a picture or graphic image,
- a chart/exhibit format, which requires the candidate to read the information in the chart/exhibit in order to answer the item, and
- a drag-and-drop question type that requires a candidate to rank order or move options to provide the correct answer.

Any of the above item formats, including standard multiple-choice items, may include charts, tables or graphic images. Students are allowed to use an on-screen optional calculator during the licensure examination.

The intent of this variety of testing formats is to assess nursing content areas with greater accuracy. For example, having the student type in an answer to a calculation question may assess drug dosage calculation competency more accurately than having the student choose from among four given answers.

The CD includes a module entitled Preparation for NCLEX, which has 50 dosage calculation questions presented in various testing formats. This will provide the student with additional practice with the content covered in *Calculating Drug Dosages: An Interactive Approach to Learning Nursing Math*, as well as practice with the different test item formats included in the NCLEX. The pop-up calculator is available for student use.

This Instructor's Guide includes sample questions that can be given to the students to explain the different NCLEX testing formats. These questions, which can be used in a dosage calculation class, clinical conference, or an NCLEX preparation seminar, provide one more way to ensure your students' success on the licensure exam.

STANDARD, FOUR OPTION, MULTIPLE CHOICE QUESTIONS:

1. The physician orders an IV of 1 liter ½ NS at 80 mL / hour for a newly admitted patient. The nurse sets up the IV with an IV tubing labeled 15 gtt / mL. The nurse is correct to time the flow rate of the gravity IV to:
   - ○ a.   20 mL / hr
   - ○ b.   20 gtt / min
   - ○ c.   250 mL / hr
   - ○ d.   250 gtt / min

2. The patient calls the nurse and states that he has chest pain. The nurse checks the doctor's medication orders in the chart and verifies the order for nitroglycerine 0.6 mg SL tablet p.r.n. chest pain q.5 minutes x 3 doses. The following forms of nitroglycerine are available:

Nitroglycerine 9 mg extended-release tablet Lot: ABC Exp: 02/09/xx	Nitroglycerine 6.5 mg extended-release capsule Lot: ACS Exp: 02/15/xx
Nitroglycerine 0.3 mg sublingual tablet Lot: BES Exp: 04/21/xx	Nitroglycerine 0.4 mg sublingual tablet Lot: TRX Exp: 07/17/xx

   The nurse is correct to administer:
   - ○ a.   2/3 of a 9 mg extended-release tablet
   - ○ b.   One 6.5 mg extended-release capsule
   - ○ c.   Two 0.3 mg sublingual tablets
   - ○ d.   2/3 of a 0.4 mg sublingual tablet

MULTIPLE CHOICE QUESTIONS THAT REQUIRE MORE THAN ONE RESPONSE:

3. The nurse is instructing a new nursing assistant about I & O for the assigned patients. The nurse should include which of the following examples of intake that should be measured? Select all that apply:

   ☐ a. 1 cup of coffee
   ☐ b. 6 ounces of apple juice
   ☐ c. 4 teaspoons of scrambled eggs
   ☐ d. 1/3 cup of orange-flavored gelatin
   ☐ e. a 90 mL lime popsicle

4. The nurse is preparing to administer 31 units of insulin to the patient. Which of the following syringes could the nurse choose to accurately administer this dose of insulin? Select all that apply:

   ☐ a. tuberculin syringe with mL markings
   ☐ b. 1 cc standard insulin syringe with even markings
   ☐ c. 1 cc insulin syringe with even and odd markings
   ☐ d. 1/2 cc insulin syringe
   ☐ e. 3/10 cc insulin syringe

FILL-IN-THE-BLANK QUESTIONS:

5. The doctor orders amiodarone 0.5 mg / min IV for a patient with ventricular arrythmias. The pharmacy sends a 500 mL bag of D5W with 900 mg amiodarone added. What rate of administration will the nurse set on the IV pump (mL / hr) to correctly administer the ordered dose?
   ANSWER:

   _____

6. The nurse is preparing to give a dose of oral antibiotic medication to a 18-month-old patient. The accurate, ordered dose is contained in 0.55 mL of medication. What type of medication administration equipment is best to administer the antiobiotic to the child accurately?
   ANSWER:

   _____

QUESTIONS THAT REQUIRE IDENTIFICATION OF AN AREA ON A PICTURE OR GRAPHIC IMAGE:

7. The day shift nurse learns in the change-of-shift report that the patient's IV of D5/0.45NS has 975 mL remaining at 0600. The IV is ordered to infuse at 75 mL / hr. At 1400, the nurse calculates IV intake for the patient. Put a line on the IV bag to identify the level of IV fluid remaining at 1400.

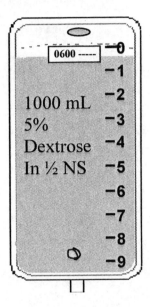

8. The nurse is calculating the body surface area (BSA) of an infant who weighs 16 pounds. Put an "x" on the line that identifies the BSA of the child in m^2 on the West Nomogram below.

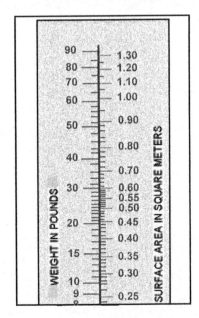

QUESTIONS IN A CHART/EXHIBIT FORMAT:

9. The nurse is preparing to administer a morning insulin dose to a diabetic patient. The patient's 0700 finger stick blood glucose result is 235 mg / dL. The doctor's orders for insulin and hospital protocol for diabetic sliding scale are as follows:

Date	Physician's Orders
	1. Regular insulin 4 units with NPH insulin 12 units q.AM.
	2. Moderate sliding scale per hospital protocol.
	Signature MD
	PATIENT'S NAME ID ************

DIABETIC SLIDING SCALE PROTOCOL			
Blood glucose (mg / dL)	Mild dose (Regular insulin)	Moderate dose (Regular insulin)	Aggressive dose (Regular insulin)
Less than 60	SEE HYPOGLYCEMIC PROTOCOL		
60 – 150	0 units	0 units	0 units
151 – 200	0 units	3 units	4 units
201 – 250	2 units	5 units	6 units
251 – 300	4 units	7 units	10 units
301 – 350	8 units	10 units	12 units
Greater than 350	10 units	12 units	15 units
	AND CALL PHYSICIAN		

The total amount of insulin that the nurse would administer at 0700 is:

- ○ a. 5 units
- ○ b. 16 units
- ○ c. 18 units
- ○ d. 21 units

10. The doctor orders carvedilol 12.5 mg for a patient with congestive heart failure. The pharmacy sends the following medication:

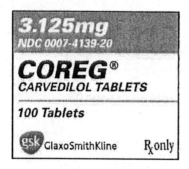

3.125mg
NDC 0007-4139-20

COREG®
CARVEDILOL TABLETS

100 Tablets

gsk GlaxoSmithKline   R only

How many tablet(s) should the nurse administer?
ANSWER:

_____

DRAG-AND-DROP QUESTIONS THAT REQUIRE RANKING OR MOVING OPTIONS TO PROVIDE THE CORRECT ANSWER:

11. The clinic nurse is preparing to teach a patient about reconstitution of a powdered IV medication, for administration through a peripherally inserted central catheter at home. The nurse writes the steps of the reconstitution process for the patient to use at home. Place all of the steps listed below in descending chronological order (1st step to last step). Use all of the options.

<table>
<tr><th>UNORDERED OPTIONS</th><th></th><th>ORDERED OPTIONS</th></tr>
<tr><td>Insert diluent into the vial of powder.</td><td rowspan="5">⇨ ⇦</td><td rowspan="5"></td></tr>
<tr><td>Withdraw 1 mL of the mixed solution.</td></tr>
<tr><td>Shake the vial.</td></tr>
<tr><td>Insert 1 mL air into the vial of diluent.</td></tr>
<tr><td>Withdraw 1 mL of diluent.</td></tr>
</table>

12. The nurse is reviewing needle sizes in preparation for a hospital competency review. Put the following in order, from the smallest gauge needle to the largest gauge needle (for example: a, b, c, d). Use all of the options.
    a. 18 G
    b. 22 G
    c. 27 G
    d. 25 G

    TYPE THE ANSWER IN THE BOX BELOW:

FOCUS ON SAFETY

TO THE INSTRUCTOR:

In 1999, the Institute of Medicine (IOM) published *To Err is Human: Building a Safer Health System.* This report called attention to the error-prone medication system present in most healthcare organizations. The IOM report emphasized that errors were a result of problems in the entire medication use system (including prescribing, communication of orders, medication labels and packaging, dispensing, administration, education, and monitoring of medications), and not just due to individual carelessness or error.

The Joint Commission on Accreditation of Healthcare Organizations (JCAHO), the Institute for Safe Medication Practices (ISMP), and other professional organizations continue to publish guidelines and standards to promote safety in all aspects of patient care, including medication administration. These guidelines include JCAHO's National Patient Safety Goals and the "Do-Not-Use" lists of unacceptable and dangerous abbreviations.

The second edition of *Calculating Drug Doses: An Interactive Approach to Learning Nursing Math* includes new Focus on Safety exercises throughout the CD. These exercises present common clinical situations related to safe administration of medications. Students are asked to make a clinical judgment and to give a rationale for their thinking and planned actions. Focus on Safety exercises provide the student with practice in critical thinking and help students correlate math calculation skills with real-world clinical situations related to medication safety.

Focus on Safety highlights are also found in the revised Student Workbook.

This revision of the Instructor's Guide includes two worksheets with Focus on Safety situations that can be given to the students to stimulate critical thinking during a clinical conference, seminar, or large classroom discussion.

Name: _____

Date: _____

Worksheet:
Making Clinical Judgments in Medication Administration

Read each situation, and then make a clinical judgment. Provide a rationale for your decision or action:

1.

Date	Physician's Orders
3/18	Acetaminophen 325 mg give ii q.4-6hr. p.r.n. temperature greater than 101° F.

Signature MD

Patient's name
ID **********

SITUATION:
The patient complains of pain in her joints. She tells the nurse that she always takes two acetaminophen tablets for joint pain at home. The nurse checks the MD order. What is the best action for the nurse?

a. call the MD to clarify the order.

b. administer two 325 mg tabs of acetaminophen.

c. call the pharmacist.

Rationale / Discussion:

2.

Date	Physician's Orders
7/21	1. N.P.O. 2. Insert NG tube. X-ray for placement. 3. Once placement confirmed, resume previous medications. 4. KCl 40 mEq per NG at 4 PM.

Signature MD

7/21 1130 noted, J.D., R.N

Patient's name
ID **********

KCl 20 mEq
[extended-release tablet]

Lot: APR   Exp: 08/15/xx

SITUATION:
The PM shift nurse checks the MD's orders from the previous shift, and the patient's medication drawer. At 1545, radiology calls to confirm correct placement of the nasogastric tube. At 1600, the nurse crushes and administers two KCl 20 mEq tablets per NG tube. The nurse's action:

a. correctly follows the MD orders because . . .

b. is incorrect, and requires further action

Rationale / Discussion:

3.

SITUATION:
Nurse A checks the morning dose of insulin with Nurse B, by showing Nurse B the following insulin syringe. The order is for regular insulin 17 units and NPH insulin 11 units before breakfast. Did Nurse A follow the correct procedure for checking insulin dosage?

a. yes, because . .

b. no, because . . .

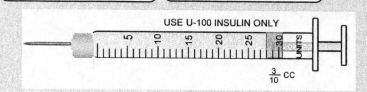

USE U-100 INSULIN ONLY

$\frac{3}{10}$ CC

Rationale / Discussion:

4.

Medication Administration Record			
Date	Medication Order	Time	Initials
10/7	Ibuprofen 400 mg p.o. q.6h. ATC	~~0400~~ ~~1000~~ 1600 2200	JB RN TT RN
10/7	Morphine sulfate 5 mg IV q.4h. PRN severe pain (greater than 7/10)	0800 1210	TT RN TT RN
		Patient X ID ********	

SITUATION:
The PM shift nurse checks the medication administration record at 1600, to determine when Patient X is due for pain medication. The patient is complaining of pain of "8" on a scale of 1 – 10. The nurse is most correct in giving Patient X:

a. IV morphine sulfate

b. PO ibuprofen

c. IV morphine sulfate and PO ibuprofen

Rationale / Discussion:

5.

SITUATION:
The order is for amoxicillin suspension 2 g q.8h. for a patient with a bacterial infection. The medication comes from the pharmacy in a bottle labeled 400 mg / 5 mL. Did the nurse pour the correct amount of amoxicillin suspension into the medicine cup?

a. yes, because . .

b. no, because . . .

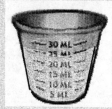

30 ML
25 ML
20 ML
15 ML
10 ML
5 ML

Rationale / Discussion:

Worksheet:
Making Clinical Judgments in IV Administration

Read each situation, and then make a clinical judgment. Provide a rationale for your decision or action:

1.

High Alert

epinephrine
(e-pi-**nef**-rin)

CLASSIFICATION(S):
Therapeutic: antiasthmatics, bronchodilators, vasopressors
Pharmacologic: adrenergics

IMPLEMENTATION
High Alert: Patient harm or fatalities have occurred from medication errors with epinephrine. Epinephrine is available in various concentrations, strengths, and percentages. . . .
 IV: Dilute 1 mg (1mL) of 1:1000 solution in at least 10 mL of 0.9% NaCl for injection, to prepare a 1:10,000 solution. . . .
 Direct IV: Administer each 1 mg (10 mL) of 1:10,000 solution over at least 1 min; more rapid administration may be used during cardiac resuscitation.

SITUATION:
The physician orders 1:10,000 epinephrine 0.2 mg IVP now for a patient with a severe anaphylactic reaction to a bee sting. The nurse looks up the medication prior to administration and decides to give it over 1 minute. This rate of administration for the ordered dose of epinephrine is:

a. **too rapid, because . .**

b. **too slow, because . .**

c. **correct, because . . .**

Rationale / Discussion:

2.

Date	Physician's Orders
3/14 0900	1. Start IV with 500 mL NS at 30 mL / hr.
	2. Infuse 2 units packed red blood cells over five hours.
	3. Repeat Hgb at 4 PM.
	Signature MD

Patient's name
ID **********

SITUATION:
The nurse begins the first unit of packed red blood cells (PRBC) at 0930. Each unit of PRBC contains 250 mL. The blood tubing has a drop factor of 10 gtt / mL. The nurse sets the infusion of PRBC at 17 gtt / min. The nurse has:

a. **correctly set the rate of the blood infusion.**

b. **made an error in setting the rate of the blood infusion.**

Rationale / Discussion:

3.

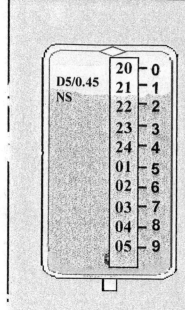

D5/0.45 NS

20	–	0
21	–	1
22	–	2
23	–	3
24	–	4
01	–	5
02	–	6
03	–	7
04	–	8
05	–	9

<u>SITUATION:</u>
At 1700, the nurse starts an IV of 1 L D5/0.45 NS with 30 mEq KCl, to infuse at 100 mL / hr. The IV infiltrates at 1830 and is restarted at 2000. The nurse relabels the IV at 2000, and the IV infuses well though the remainder of the evening shift (1500 – 2300). Did the nurse correctly label the IV bag after the IV was restarted?

a. yes, because . . .

b. no, because . . .

Rationale / Discussion:

4.

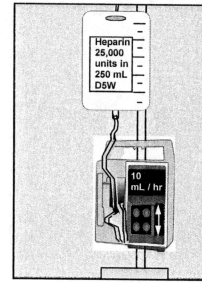

Heparin 25,000 units in 250 mL D5W

10 mL / hr

<u>SITUATION:</u>
The nurse hears in change of shift report that the patient's IV heparin is infusing at 900 units per hour via an infusion pump. The nurse checks the IV during the morning assessment. The patient's IV is infusing:

a. at the correct rate . . .

b. too slowly . . .

c. too rapidly . . .

Rationale / Discussion:

5.

INTAKE AND OUTPUT RECORD				
Date	Time	Intake		Output
		IV	PO	
12/7	0000 to 0700		250	350
	0700 to 1500	950	680	990
Total			Patient H ID *******	

<u>SITUATION:</u>
An IV is infusing at 125 mL / hr from 0700 to 1000. At 1000, the physician lowers the rate to 75 mL / hr. The patient receives the following IVPB medications: vancomycin 1 g in 100 mL NS q.8h. and pantoprazole 80 mg in 100 mL at 1100 and 2300. Has the day shift nurse correctly entered the patient's IV intake on the I & O record?

a. yes

b. no

Rationale / Discussion:

Name: _____

Date: _____

Basic Math Diagnostic Exam

Score_____

INSTRUCTIONS: Solve the following problems. Reduce all fractions to the lowest terms. Show all work in the space provided. Write your answer on the answer line.
Questions 1 – 20 are worth 4 points each. Questions 21 – 30 are worth 2 points each.

ADDITION:

1. $121 + 5 + 4,795 + 12 + 13,274 =$ _____

2. $34.88 + 3640 + 7 + 0.41 =$ _____

3. $46 + 0.3053 + 973.70 + 3,034.08 =$ _____

4. $18 \ 2/9 + 5/3 + 4/12 =$ _____

5.   6 1/5 + 4 2/3 + 1/2 =   _____

SUBTRACTION:

6.   32,363 − 7,895 =   _____

7.   4 − 0.824 =   _____

8.   42.908 − 2.59 =   _____

9.   11 3/8 − 4 6/10 =   _____

10. 5 3/4 − 2 4/5 =   _____

MULTIPLICATION:

11.   3752 x 406 =   _____

12.   4 2/7 x 1/2 =   _____

13.   3 1/3 x 1 5/6 =   _____

14.   25 2/5 x 5 =   _____

15.   35.005 x 1.05 =   _____

DIVISION: Work division problems 3 places to the right of the decimal point. Round the final answer to the hundredths place (2 places to the right of the decimal point).

16. $452 \div 12 =$ _____

17. $5.60 \div 14 =$ _____

18. $4\ 1/5 \div 1/75 =$ _____

19. $4\ 1/4 \div 1\ 1/2 =$ _____

20. $2\ 1/5 \div 3 =$ _____

ROMAN NUMERALS: Change the following to Arabic numbers or Roman numerals.

21.   26 = _____   22.   47 = _____   23.   90 = _____   24.   75 = _____

25.   39 = _____   26.   LIV = _____   27.   MM = _____   28.   XIII = _____

29.   VSS = _____   30.   LXXXIV = _____

Competency Exam # 1

Score_____

INSTRUCTIONS: Solve the following problems. Show all work in the space provided. Round answers to the hundredths place (2 places to the right of the decimal) unless otherwise instructed. Write your answer on the answer line. Each problem is worth 4 points.

1.   Use the drug label to fill in the following information.

FOR ORAL USE ONLY.
STORAGE
Before Reconstitution:
Store below 86°F (30°C).
After Reconstitution:
Store suspension between 41°F (5°C) and
86°F (30°C). Protect from freezing.
SHAKE WELL BEFORE EACH USE.
DISCARD UNUSED PORTION AFTER 2 WEEKS.
MIXING DIRECTIONS
Tap bottle lightly to loosen powder. Add 24 mL
of distilled water or Purified Water (USP) to the
bottle. Shake well.
DOSAGE AND USE
See accompanying prescribing information.
This package contains 350 mg fluconazole in a
natural orange-flavored mixture.*

NDC 0049-3440-19
35 mL when reconstituted

DIFLUCAN®
(Fluconazole
for Oral Suspension)

ORANGE FLAVORED

10 mg/mL

when reconstituted

Pfizer Roerig
Division of Pfizer Inc, NY, NY 10017

_____
Trade Name

_____
Generic Name

_____
Dosage Strength

**Ordered: Fluconazole 0.05 g p.o. daily.
How many tsp will the nurse give?**

_____

2.   **A patient weighs 68 kg. How many lb does the patient weigh?**

_____

3.   **The physician orders levothyroxine 0.3 mg p.o. daily. The pharmacy sends levothyroxine 150 mcg / tablet. How many tablet(s) will the nurse administer?**

_____

4. The order is for Heparin 4000 units subcut daily. The pharmacy sends a prefilled cartridge of heparin. How many mL will the nurse administer?

_____

Shade in the prefilled cartridge with the ordered dose.

1/2   1   1 1/2   2 mL

5000 units / mL   HEPARIN

5. The patient is n.p.o. for breakfast and lunch and is started on a clear liquid diet for dinner. For dinner, the patient took 6 ounces of broth, 4 T of JELL-O®, and ½ cup of tea. At 1830, the patient vomited 220 mL of fluid. An IV of 1 L D5/0.45 NS q.8h. was started at 1900. The patient voided 125 mL at 1930 and 270 mL at 2200. At the end of the shift, the nurse emptied 60 mL from the patient's wound drainage device. What is the patient's 8-hour I & O (starting at 1500 and ending at 2300)?

I _____

O _____

How much IV credit will the nurse give the next shift at 2300?

_____

What is the flow rate of the IV if the nurse uses a microdrip tubing set?

_____

6. The order is for methylprednisolone 120 mg IM daily for 7 days. The nurse has a vial of methylprednisolone labeled 80 mg / mL How many mL will the nurse administer?

_____

7. The physician orders a loading dose of esmolol hydrochloride 28 mg IV push for a patient with a cardiac dysrhythmia. The pharmacy sends the following vial. How many mL of esmolol will the patient receive?

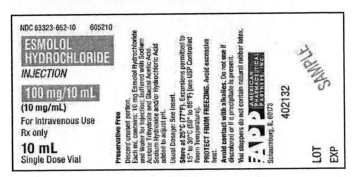

_____

The nurse decides to dilute the medication in 5 mL normal saline before administering it to the patient. Shade in the total number of mL the nurse will administer (esmolol and normal saline).

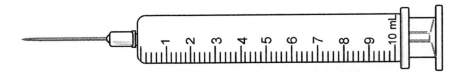

8. The patient is to receive 1 unit whole blood. The unit (475 mL) is to infuse over 2.5 hours. A blood tubing (10 gtt / mL) is used for the infusion. What is the flow rate for the whole blood?

_____

9. A patient with CHF has an order for IV theophylline 300 mg in 50 mL D5W over 30 minutes, followed by maintenance dose of IV theophylline to infuse at 20 mg / hr. The patient weighs 68 kg. The following is an excerpt from the drug reference book about theophylline. Calculate whether the ordered doses are safe doses.

theophylline
(thee-**off**-i-lin)

CLASSIFICATION(S):
Therapeutic: bronchodilators
Pharmacologic: xanthines

ROUTE AND DOSAGE:
IV (Adults): *Loading dose—*
4.7 mg / kg, then
0.55 mg / kg / hr for 12 hr,
then 0.36 mg/ kg/ hr
maintenance infusion rate.
IV (Adults with CHF):
Loading dose—4.7 mg / kg,
then 0.39 mg / kg / hr for 12
hr, then 0.08 – 0.16 mg/ kg/ hr
maintenance infusion rate.

The safe loading dose of theophylline for this patient is:

_____

Is the loading dose ordered for this patient safe?

_____

The safc maintenance dose of theophylline for this patient is:

_____

Is the maintenance dose ordered for this patient safe?

_____

10. The patient is to receive an enteral tube feeding of 1/4-strength Nepro® to infuse at 75 mL / hr through a PEG tube. At the bedside is an 8 oz can of Nepro. How many mL of water will the nurse add to the Nepro to make the correct concentration of solution?

_____

11. At 1500, the start of the shift, the patient has 700 mL of D5W infusing at 40 mL / hr. The IV infiltrates at 1800 and is restarted at 2030 at 80 mL / hr per MD order. Beginning with the amount of IV fluid left at 1800, calculate the infusion time for this IV.

_____

Calculate the completion time.   _____

12. Midazolam hydrochloride 1.5 mg is ordered for a patient prior to a procedure. The drug is available in the following vial. How many mL will the nurse administer?

_____

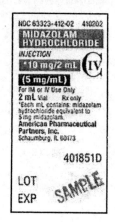

Shade in the most appropriate syringe with the desired dose.

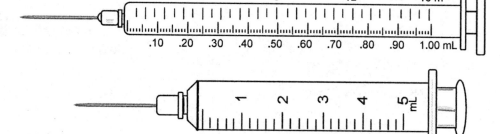

13. Amikacin 275 mg IV is ordered. The nurse has the following vial. How many mL will the nurse administer to give the ordered dose?

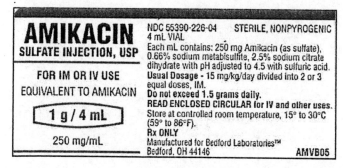

_____

14. The patient is on strict I & O. An IV of D5W is infusing at 42 mL / hr into one lumen of the patient's triple-lumen central line. At 0700, 900 mL is left in the bag. Total parenteral nutrition (TPN) is infusing into another lumen of the central line at 50 mL / hr. At 0700, 800 mL remains in the TPN bag. The nurse hangs a 500 mL bottle of fat emulsion at 42 mL / hr into the TPN line, at 1000. At 1100, the patient vomits 125 mL of yellowish fluid. The patient voids 175 mL at 0900, 375 mL at 1200, and 225 mL at 1400. At the end of the shift, the nurse empties 10 mL from the patient's wound drainage device # 1 and 50 mL from drainage device # 2. What is the patient's 8-hour I & O (0700 to 1500)?

I _____

O _____

How much credit from the fat emulsion will the nurse give to the next shift at 1500?

_____

How much credit from the TPN will the nurse give to the next shift at 1500?

_____

15. The order is for 1 L of D5/0.45 NS to infuse over 12 hours. Calculate the mL / hr.

_____

The nurse uses IV tubing labeled 12 gtt / mL. Calculate the flow rate.

_____

16. Gemcitabine 200 mg IV is ordered for the patient. The pharmacy sends the following vial. Use the label to calculate the following:

Rx *Lilly*

GEMZAR®
Gemcitabine HCl
For Injection

200 mg
equivalent to base

For I.V. use only
Sterile Single Use Vial

DO NOT REFRIGERATE

Rx only

Storage: Prior to and after re-constitution, store at controlled room temperature 20° to 25°C (68° to 77°F) [See USP].

To reconstitute: Add 5 mL of 0.9% Sodium Chloride In-jection (without preserva-tives) to make a solution containing 38 mg/mL. Shake to dissolve.

Administer solution within 24 hours. Discard unused portion.

To prepare I.V. solution—See accompanying literature.

Amount of diluent_____

Type of diluent_____

Dosage strength_____

Give_____ mL

17. **Ordered:**
    a. 1000 mL D5/0.45 NS with 20 mEq KCl at 75 mL / hr.
    b. Every shift, replace NG drainage of previous shift, mL for mL, with 2nd IV of 500 mL LR.
    c. Total hourly IV fluid not to exceed 125 mL / hr.

    The patient had a NG output of 225 mL from the previous shift. How long will it take to replace the NG output?

    _____

    If the replacement IV is started at 1600, what time with the replacement infusion be completed?

    _____

18. The nurse hangs an IV of 500 mL 0.45% NS at 2300. The IV is to infuse at 50 mL / hr. Label the flowmeter q.2h., including the starting and the completion times.

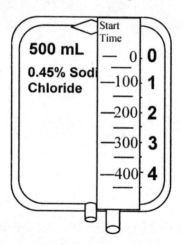

19. The order is for dobutamine 60 mg / hr for a patient who weighs 242 lb. An IV of 250 mg of dobutamine in 500 mL D5W is infusing at 150 mL / hr. The drug reference book states that the adult dosage range for dobutamine is 2 – 20 mcg / kg / min.

    Is the ordered dose a safe dose for this patient?

    _____

    Is the setting on the IV pump correct?

    _____

20. The nurse is to give fentanyl 75 mcg IM to a preoperative patient one hour before surgery. Fentanyl is available in a vial labeled 0.05 mg per mL. How many mL will the nurse give to the patient?

    _____

21. The patient has 925 mL of D5LR remaining at 1500, the start of the evening shift. The IV is infusing at 75 mL / hr. At 1800, the MD ordered the IV to infuse at 125 mL / hr for 2 hours, then to decrease the rate to 100 mL / hr. Label the flowmeter, starting with the amount of IV fluid left after the 2-hour hydration. Shade in the amount left at 2200.

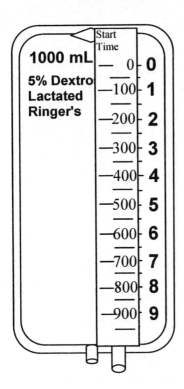

Completion time: _____

22. The doctor orders hydromorphone 2000 mcg IVP q.3h. for pain. Hyrdromorphone 3 mg / mL is available. How many mL of hydromorphone will the nurse administer?

_____

The nurse looks up hydromorphone in the drug reference book. The following information is listed for hydromorphone:

High Alert

Hydormorphone
(hye-droe-**mor**-fone)

IMPLEMENTATION
- **Direct IV:** Dilute with at least 5 mL of sterile water or 0.9% NaCl for injection.
- *Rate*: Administer slowly, at a rate not to exceed 2 mg over 3 – 5 minutes.
- *High Alert*: Rapid administration may lead to increased respiratory depression, hypotension, and circulatory collapse.

What is the rate of administration for the ordered dose of hydromorphone?

_____

23. A child with leukemia has an order for doxorubicin HCl 35 mg IV. The child weighs 70 pounds and has a body surface area of 1.10 m². The drug reference book has the following information about doxorubicin:

> **High Alert**
>
> **doxorubicin hydrochloride**
> (dox-oh-**roo**-bi-sin hye-droe-**klor**-ide
>
> **ROUTE AND DOSAGE:**
> **IV (Children):** 30 mg / m² / day for 3 days every 4 wk.

What is the maximum safe dose based on the drug literature for this child?

_____

Is the ordered dose safe for this child?

_____

24. The patient has the following insulin orders:

> 1. Humulin 70/30 23 units at 0730.
> 2. Humulin Regular insulin subcut q.i.d. a.c. & bedtime:
>   Give 2 units for BS 150 – 175 mg / dL.
>   Give 5 units for BS 176 – 225 mg / dL.
>   Give 10 units for BS 226 – 260 mg / dL.
>   Call MD BS greater than 260 mg / dL.

The nurse is told in morning report that the patient's blood sugar at 0630 was 226 mg / dL. Based on the orders above, what is the total amount of insulin that the patient will receive before breakfast?

_____

Shade in the most appropriate syringe below with the total amount of insulin given.

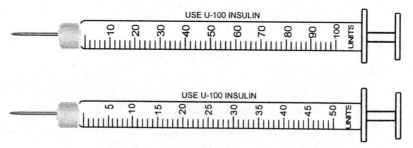

25. Ketoconazole 200 mg is ordered. Available is a bottle labeled ketoconazole oral suspension 0.1 g / 5 mL. How many mL will the nurse administer?

_____

Name: _____

Date: _____

Competency Exam #2

Score _____

INSTRUCTIONS: Solve the following problems. Show all work in the space provided. Round answers to the hundredths place (2 places to the right of the decimal) unless otherwise instructed. Write your answer on the answer line. Each problem is worth 4 points.

1. The patient is returned to the unit at 1000 after removal of a bladder tumor. He has a continuous bladder irrigation infusing at 175 mL / hr. He starts on clear liquids for lunch, and has 1 cup of tea, 6 ounces of chicken broth, and 200 mL of lemon-lime soda. His IV is infusing at 150 mL / hr until 1400, when the physician lowers the rate to 100 mL / hr. The nurse hangs an IVPB of cefoxitin 1 g in 50 mL D5W at 1300, and a second IVPB of famotidine 20 mg in 50 mL D5W at 1400. At the end of the shift, the nursing assistant reports that he has emptied 1500 mL from the patient's indwelling catheter bag. What is the patient's I & O from 1000 to 1500?

   I _____

   O _____

2. Use the drug label to fill in the following information.

   ```
   NDC 0409-2266-02
   2 mL Single-dose Discard unused portion
   Alfentanil Inj., USP
   1000 mcg/2 mL (500 mcg/mL)
   May be habit forming.    ℞ only
   For I.V. use.
   Hospira, Inc., Lake Forest, IL 60045 USA
   ```

   Total amount in vial
   _____

   Controlled substance?
   _____

   Dosage Strength
   _____

   If the patient is to receive an IV dose of 1 mg, how many mL of alfentanil will be administered?   _____

3. A patient weighs 176 pounds. How many kg does the patient weigh?

   _____

4. The physician orders 1 unit fresh frozen plasma for a patient with disseminated intravascular coagulation. The unit (300 mL) is to infuse over 2 hours. A blood tubing (10 gtt / mL) is used for the infusion. What is the flow rate for the fresh frozen plasma?

_____

5. The physician writes the following order for a patient on mechanical ventilation: midazolam 3 mg IV loading dose now, followed by 3 mg in 10 minutes x 3, until adequate sedation is achieved. Follow with an infusion of 500 mL D5W with 250 mg of midazolam @ 10 mg / hr. The patient weighs 85 kg. The following is an excerpt from the drug reference book about midazolam HCl. Calculate whether the ordered doses are safe.

High Alert

midazolam
(mid-**ay**-zoe-lam)

Anti-anxiety agents, sedative / hypnotics

Sedation in critical care settings:
IV (Adults): 10 – 50 mcg / kg (0.5 – 4 mg in most adults) initially if a loading dose is required; may repeat q.10 – 15 min until desired effect is obtained; may be followed by infusion at 20 – 100 mcg / kg / hr (1 – 7 mg / hr in most adults).

The safe loading dose of midazolam for this patient is:

_____

Is the ordered loading dose safe?

_____

The maximum infusion rate of midazolam for this patient is:

_____

Is the ordered infusion rate safe?

_____

6. The patient is to receive an enteral tube feeding of ¾-strength Jevity® at 50 mL / hr through a PEG tube. The can of Jevity contains 237 mL. How many mL of water will the nurse add to the Jevity to make the correct concentration of solution?

_____

7. At 1700, 1000 mL D5/0.225 NS with 20 mEq KCl is started. The IV is to infuse at 60 mL / hr. Calculate the infusion time for this IV.

_____

Calculate the completion time.

_____

8.   The order is for Heparin 7500 units subcut daily. The following vials of heparin are available. Circle the most appropriate vial of heparin for the nurse to use, then calculate the number of mL that the nurse will administer.

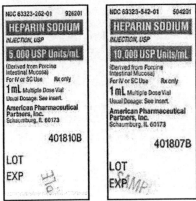

_____

Shade in the syringe with the ordered dose.

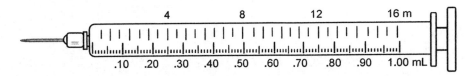

9.   The patient is n.p.o. An IV of 1 L D5/0.45 NS is infusing at 60 mL / hr into one lumen of the patient's triple-lumen central line. At 0700, 850 mL is left in the bag. Total parenteral nutrition (TPN) is infusing into another lumen of the central line at 42 mL / hr. At 0700, 450 mL remain in the bottle. The orders for IVPB include two medications during the day shift: one in 50 mL D5W and one in 100 mL D5W. At 0930, the patient vomited 50 mL of yellow fluid. The patient voided 275 mL at 0830, 425 mL at 1130, and 120 mL at 1400. At the end of the shift, the nurse emptied 45 mL from the patient's wound drainage device. What is the patient's 8-hour I & O (starting at 0700 and ending at 1500)?

I _____

O _____

How much credit from the primary IV will the nurse give to the next shift at 1500?

_____

How much credit from the TPN will the nurse give to the next shift at 1500?

_____

10. The doctor orders amiodarone 360 mg in 250 mL D5W at 1 mg / minute for a patient with ventricular dysrhythmias. Calculate the mL / hour for the infusion.

_____

11. The doctor leaves the following order: Measure patient's multiple decubitus ulcers on right leg and hip and chart measurements. The nurse measures the following:
right ankle—30 mm circular, right lateral calf—25.4 mm irregular, right posterior calf—250 mm linear, right hip—32.5 mm circular. Calculate each measurement in cm.

ankle _____

lateral calf _____

posterior calf _____

hip _____

12. Ordered:
    a. 500 mL D5/0.33 NS with 10 mEq KCl at 65 mL / hr.
    b. Every shift, replace NG drainage of previous shift, mL for mL, with 2nd IV of D5/0.45 NS with 20 mEq KCl per 500 mL.
    c. Total hourly IV fluid not to exceed 90 mL / hr.

    The patient had a NG output of 180 mL from the previous shift. How long will it take to replace the NG output?

    _____

    If the replacement IV is started at 0730, what time will the replacement infusion be completed?

    _____

13. The order is for 2 units of whole blood (500 mL each) to infuse over 6 hours. The available blood administration set has a drop factor of 10 gtt / mL. What is the flow rate for the 2 units of blood?

    _____

14. The nurse hangs an IV of 500 mL 0.45% NS at 1500. The IV is to infuse at 25 mL / hr. Label the flowmeter q.2h., including the starting and the completion times.

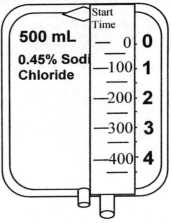

15. An infusion of penicillin G potassium 11 million units in 1 L of D5W is ordered. Use the label to calculate the the desired amount to add to the 1 L of D5W.

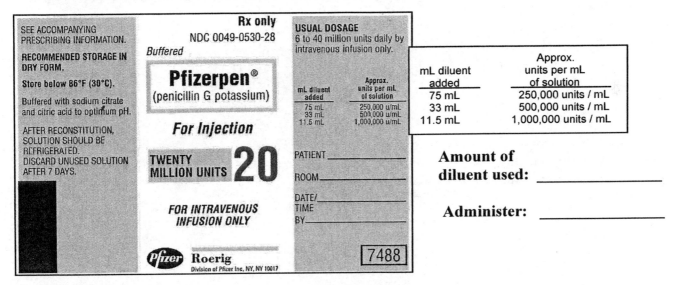

mL diluent added	Approx. units per mL of solution
75 mL	250,000 units / mL
33 mL	500,000 units / mL
11.5 mL	1,000,000 units / mL

Amount of diluent used: _____

Administer: _____

16. The patient's discharge orders include nitroglycerin ointment 30 mg topically q.8h., to prevent chest pain. The pharmacy sends a tube of transdermal nitroglycerin ointment labeled 15 mg = 1 inch. How many inches of nitroglycerin ointment will the nurse instruct the patient to take?

_____

17. Cefaclor oral suspension 375 mg b.i.d. is ordered. The nurse calculates the dose to be 2 tsp. How many mL will the nurse administer? Fill in the desired dose in the medicine cup.

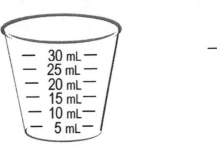

_____

18. Ranitidine 35 mg IV is ordered q.6h. How many mL will the nurse administer?

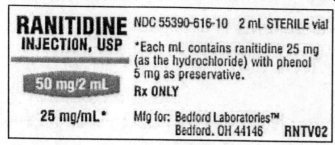

_____

Shade in the desired dose in the most appropriate syringe.

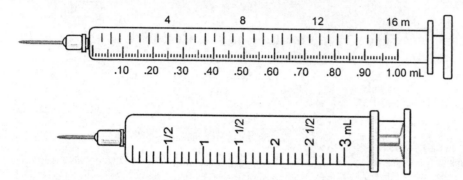

19. The doctor orders morphine sulfate 18 mg IVP q.2h., as an interval dose for a patient with spinal metastasis. The following vial of morphine sulfate is available. How many mL of morphine will the nurse administer?

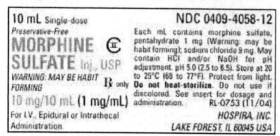

_____

The nurse looks up morphine in the drug reference book. The following information is listed for morphine:

> **High Alert**
>
> **morphine**
> (mor-feen)
>
> **IMPLEMENTATION**
> - **Direct IV: Dilute with at least 5 mL of sterile water or 0.9% NaCl for injection.**
> - _Rate: High Alert:_ **Administer 2.5 – 15 mg over 4 – 5 minutes. Rapid administration may lead to increased respiratory depression, hypotension, and circulatory collapse.**

What is the rate of administration for the ordered dose of morphine?

_____

20. The patient has 850 mL of D5LR remaining at 1500, the start of the evening shift. The IV is infusing at 75 mL / hr. At 1700, the MD ordered the IV to infuse at 150 mL / hr for 2 hours, then to decrease the rate to 100 mL / hr. Label the flowmeter, starting with the amount of IV fluid left after the 2-hour hydration. Shade in the amount left at 2200.

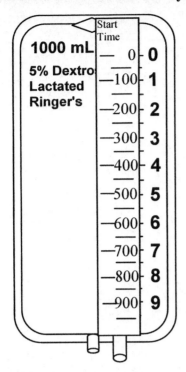

Completion time: _____

21. The patient has the following insulin orders:

> 1. Humulin 50/50 14 units at 0730.
> 2. Humulin Regular insulin q.i.d. a.c. & bedtime:
>   Give 2 units for BS > 150 < 175 mg / dL.
>   Give 5 units for BS > 176 < 225 mg / dL.
>   Give 10 units for BS > 226 < 260 mg / dL.
>   Call MD if BS > 260 mg / dL.

The nurse is told in the morning report that the patient's blood sugar at 0630 was 220 mg / dL. Based on the orders above, what is the total amount of insulin that the patient will receive before breakfast?

_____

Shade in the most appropriate syringe below with the total amount of insulin given.

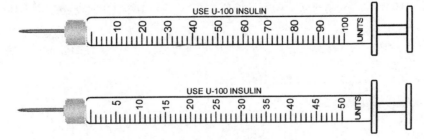

22. The patient has an IV of D5/0.225 NS infusing at 125 mL / hr at 0700, the beginning of the shift. The night shift reported that 875 mL was remaining in the IV bag at 0700. The IV infiltrated at 1000 and was restarted at 12 noon. The MD came in at 1300 and decreased the rate of the IV to 75 mL / hr. How many mL of IV fluid infused into the patient during the day shift (0700–1500)?

_____

How much is left in the IV bag at 1500?

_____

23. A child with leukemia has an order for vincristine 2 mg IV. The patient weighs 88 pounds and has a body surface area of 1.3 m². The drug reference book has the following information about vincristine:

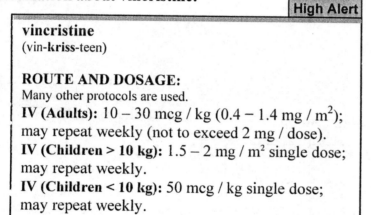

High Alert

vincristine
(vin-**kriss**-teen)

ROUTE AND DOSAGE:
Many other protocols are used.
IV (Adults): 10 – 30 mcg / kg (0.4 – 1.4 mg / m²); may repeat weekly (not to exceed 2 mg / dose).
IV (Children > 10 kg): 1.5 – 2 mg / m² single dose; may repeat weekly.
IV (Children < 10 kg): 50 mcg / kg single dose; may repeat weekly.

What is the maximum safe dose based on the drug literature for this child?

_____

Is the ordered dose safe for this child?   _____

24. The physician orders Vitamin B_{12} 1500 mcg IM subcut. The pharmacy sends an ampule labeled Vitamin B_{12} 1 mg / mL. How many mL will the nurse administer?

_____

Shade in the syringe with the desired dose.

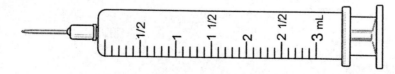

25. The order is for dopamine 8 mg / hr for a 35-year-old patient who weighs 132 pounds. The intent of the medication is to improve renal blood flow. An IV of 400 mg of dopamine in 500 mL D5W is infusing at 14 mL / hr. The drug reference book states the following about the usual adult dosages for dopamine:

dopamine
(dope-a-meen)

ROUTE AND DOSAGE:

IV (Adults): *Dopaminergic (renal vasodilation) effects*—0.5 – 3 mcg / kg / min. *Beta-adrenergic (cardiac stimulation) effects*—2 – 10 mcg / kg / min. *Alpha-adrenergic (increased peripheral vascular resistance) effects*—10 mcg / kg / min; infusion rate may be increased as needed.
IV (Children): 5 – 20 mcg / kg / min, depending on desired response (0.5 – 3 mcg / kg / min has been used to improve renal blood flow).

Is the ordered dose a safe dose for this patient?

_____

Is the setting on the IV pump correct?

_____

Worksheet: Using Decimals and Fractions in Medication Administration (p. 2)

1.   0.75   2.   0.5   3.   0.25

4.   9 tablets

5.   0.425 g
      2 tabs of 0.225 g and 1 tab of 0.2 g

6.   4.5 mg
      2 of the 3 mg capsules and 1 of the 1.5 mg capsules

Worksheet: Using Decimals in Medication Administration (p. 3)

1. The calculated dose is 2.   2. The calculated dose is 0.25.   3. The calculated dose is 0.5.

4. The calculated dose is 125.   5. The calculated dose is 0.25.

Worksheet: Rounding Decimals in Medication Administration (p. 4)

1. Thousandths place = 1.678   6. Hundredths place = 2.43

2. Hundredths place = 1.68   7. Tenths place = 2.4

3. Tenths place = 1.7   8. Whole number = 2

4. Whole number = 2   9. Tenths place = 0.5

5. Thousandths place = 2.433   10. Whole number = 2

Worksheet: Using Roman Numerals in Medication Administration (p. 5)

1. a. 1   b. 5   c. 10   d. 4
   e. 6   f. 9   g. 12   h. 3

2. 7 oz   25 oz
    2 tsp   15 tsp
    6 Tbs   4 Tbs

3. a. oz XLI   b. tsp iii   c. T i
   d. mL L   e. mL XXX   f. mL xix

4. a. mL XC   b. oz XXX   c. mL C   d. oz XV

90   Copyright © 2007, F. A. Davis Company

Worksheet: Methods of Calculation (p. 7 – 9)

1.a.
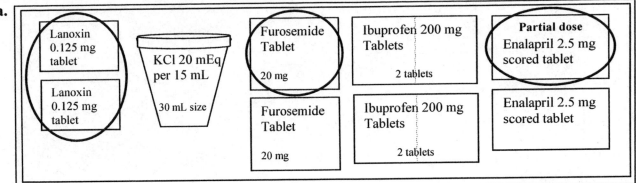

- b. **1/2 tablet**
- c. **22.5 mL**

2. **0.4 mL**

3.a. **The amoxicillin chewable tablets may be given, but the nurse needs to question whether this is the best form of drug for the individual patient.**
- b. **4 tablets**

4. **7.5 mL**

5. **1280 mg**

6. **0.375 mL (0.38 mL)**

7. **1.2 mL**

8.a.
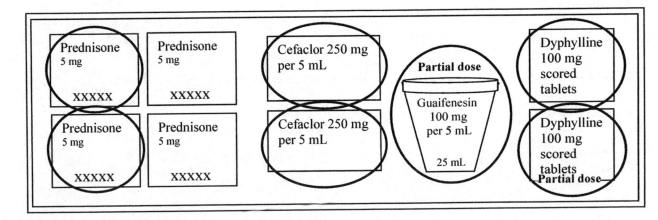

- b. **17.5 mL**
- c. **1.5 tablets**
- d. **Prednisone is not to be given on 7/24.**

9. **15 mL**

10. **0.25 mL**

Worksheet: Using the Metric System in Medication Administration (p. 11)

1. 250 mg
2. 5000 mcg
3. 2 g
4. 1,000,000 mcg
5. 2 cm

Worksheet: Using the Household System in Medication Administration (p. 12)

1. 6 tsp
2. 1 Tbs
3. 2 Tbs
4. 3 tsp
5. 12 Tbs

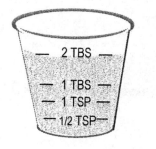
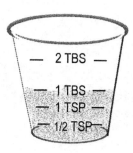
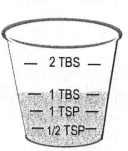

Worksheet: Converting Between Systems of Measurement in Clinical Practice (p. 13)

1. a. 500 mg   b. 250 mg
   c. 2000 mg   d. 3500 mg
   e. 0.1 mg   f. 0.75 mg

2. a. 1/2 oz   b. 1 oz
   c. 2 tsp   d. 2 Tbs
   e. 2500 mL   f. 400 mL

3. a. 182.88 cm   b. 300 mg   c. 15 mL, 3 tsp
      184.8 lb   10 mL   64 oz, 1920 mL
      0.5 cm   1000 mL   16 oz, 480 mL
      7.62 cm   300 mL
      10,000 M   15 mL
      7.5 dL   0.06 g

Worksheet: __Intake and Output (p. 15 – 16)__

1. **Yes, the charting is correct.**

2.a. **465 mL**

coffee and creamer	135 mL
bouillon	180 mL
JELL-O	90 mL
milk	60 mL
Total	465 mL

2.b. **720 mL**

coffee and creamer	270 mL
bouillon	180 mL
JELL-O	90 mL
milk	240 mL
Total	780 mL

3.

Intake and Output

	oral	IV	urine	emesis	other
7 – 3	240 90 120 240 60	600	325 190	80	Drains #1 #2 50 7
total	750	600	515	80	50 7

4.

Intake and Output

	oral	IV	urine	emesis	other
7 – 3	370	1000	cath. 475		diarrhea 120
total	370	1000	475		120
3 – 11	90	1175	cath. 350	65	
total	90	1175	350	65	
11 – 7	50	1200	375	35	90 120 60
total	50	1200	375	35	270
24-hr total	510	3375	1200	100	390

24-hour intake: 3885 mL
24-hour output: 1690 mL

5. **890 mL**

Worksheet: __Parenteral Intake (p. 17)__

1. **No, the IVPB for the 7 – 3 shift is not recorded correctly. The correct amount is 250 mL. The total 24-hour intake is 2300 mL.**
2. **700 mL**
3. **610 mL**
4. **1238 mL**

Worksheet: __Tube Feedings (p. 18 – 19)__

1. **237 mL**
2. **711 mL**
3.a. **79 mL**
  b. **316 mL**
  c. **1930**

4.a. **1000 mL**
  b. **1200 calories**
  c. **20 hours later, at 2200**
  d. **1800**
5.a. **474 mL**
  b. **700 mL**

Worksheet: **Reading Medication Labels (p. 21 – 23)**

1.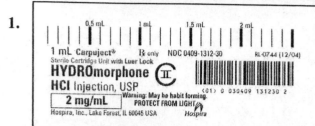

   a. ◎No   Generic name
   b. ◎Yes
   c. ◎Yes
   d. ◎Yes
   e. ◎No   1 mL is the total amount of drug

2.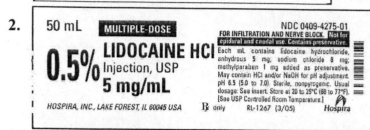

   a. ◎No   Generic name
   b. ◎Yes
   c. ◎No   Multiple-dose vial
   d. ◎Yes
   e. ◎No   Infiltration and Nerve Block

3.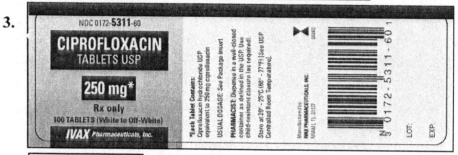

   a. ◎Yes
   b. ◎Yes
   c. ◎Yes
   d. ◎No   250 mg / tablet
   e. ◎Yes

4.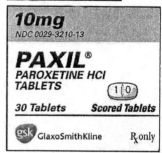

   a. ◎Yes
   b. ◎No   5 mg / 2 mL or 2.5 mg / mL
   c. ◎Yes
   d. ◎No
   e. ◎Yes

5.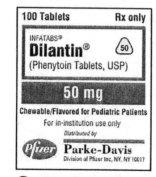

   a. ◎No   50 mg / 1 tablet

6.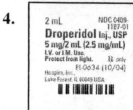

   a. ◎No   paroxetine HCl is the generic name
   b. ◎Yes
   c. ◎No   Not on the label
   d. ◎Yes
   e. ◎Yes

7.

   a. ◎Yes
   b. ◎Yes   Also 1 mg / 10 mL
   c. ◎No   Single-dose vial

8.

   a. ◎No   25 mg / tab
   b. ◎Yes

Worksheet: Introduction to Oral Medications (p. 25 – 26)

1. ☐ The medication order is transcribed incorrectly.
   The Six Rights of Administration include the correct patient. This order is transcribed on the medication record for Patient O and the order is for Patient A.

2. ☐ The medication order is transcribed incorrectly.
   The medication is to be given at bedtime. The time indicated on the medication record is 1000 or 10:00 AM.

3. ☐ The medication order is transcribed correctly.

4. ☐ The medication order is transcribed incorrectly.
   The medication is ordered q.8h. and the times on the medication record are not correct.

5. ☐ The medication order is transcribed incorrectly.
   The enteric-coated tablets may not be crushed.

6. ☐ The medication order is transcribed incorrectly.
   The medication ordered is Percocet, not Percodan.

7. ☐ The medication order is transcribed correctly.

Worksheet: Components of the Medication Order (p. 27)

1. ☐ The medication order is incorrect. The frequency of administration is missing.
   ☐ Call the MD.

2. ☐ The medication order is correct.
   ☐ Administer the medication as ordered.

3. ☐ The medication order is incorrect. The route of administration is missing.
   ☐ Call the MD.

Worksheet: Calculating Oral Drug Dosages in Medication Administration (p. 28)

1. 2 tablets

2. 2 tablets

3.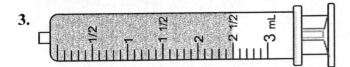

<u>**Worksheet:**</u>   **Using Syringes in Clinical Practice (p. 30 – 31)**

1. a. **b or a**   d. **a**
   b. **a**   e.   **a or b**
   c. **e or f**

2. a. **correct**
   b. **incorrect (Correct amount cannot be accurately measured in a 3 mL syringe.)**
   c. **incorrect**

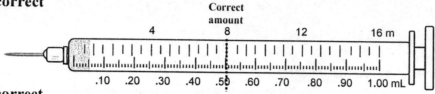

   d. **incorrect**

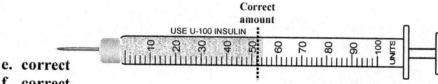

   e. **correct**
   f. **correct**
   g. **correct**

<u>**Worksheet:**</u>   **Using Needles in Clinical Practice (p. 32)**

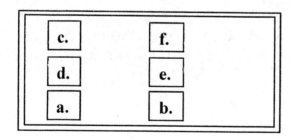

2.a. **Correct**   (A clean needle will not expose tissue to irritating medication.)
   b. **Incorrect (Massaging will cause further irritation.)**
   c. **Correct**   (Medication will have time to settle before needle is removed; Z-track technique.)
   d. **Incorrect (Injection should be given deep IM.)**

3. **Insulin syringe (The needle is permanently attached to this syringe.)**

<u>**Worksheet:**</u>   **Syringes and Needles in Clinical Practice (p. 33)**

1. a. **Standard IM:**   **3 mL 21 – 23G 1 ½"**   d. **Insulin: 3/10, 1/2, or 1 cc 28 – 31G 5/16 – 1/2"**
   b. **IM (obese):**   **3 mL 21 – 23G 2"**   e. **ID:**   **1 mL 26 – 27G 3/8"**
   c. **Subcut:**   **3 mL 25G 5/8"**   f. **IV:**   **3 – 10 mL 18 – 19G 1"**

2. **Heparin:**   **correct**
   Morphine: **correct**
   Ketorolac: **incorrect (The plunger needs to be advanced to the 2 mL line.)**

Worksheet: Parenteral Medications (p. 35 – 36)

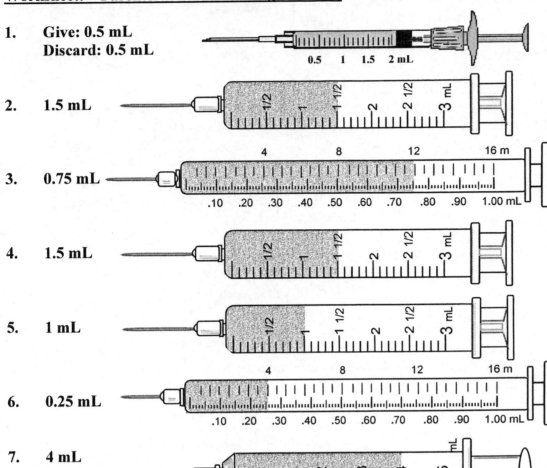

1.   Give: 0.5 mL
     Discard: 0.5 mL

2.   1.5 mL

3.   0.75 mL

4.   1.5 mL

5.   1 mL

6.   0.25 mL

7.   4 mL

Worksheet: Working With Insulin Orders (p. 37)

1.   13 units

2.   32 units

3.   2 units

4.   3 units

Worksheet: Single-Strength Reconstitution (p. 39 – 40)

1.a. Water (tap water)

b. First add approximately 58 mL. Shake vigorously. Add the remaining 29 mL; again, shake vigorously.

c. 250 mg / 5 mL

d. The total volume of the mixed medication; notice that only 87 mL of water was added. The 13 mL difference is the displacement volume of the Augmentin powder.

e. 9 mL

f. 1330 on 4/22

2.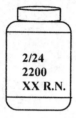

2/24
2200
XX R.N.

Date: 2/24
Time: 2200
Nurse's initials

3.a. 0.9% sodium chloride injection, USP

b. 5 mL

c. 40 mcg / mL

d. 2.5 mL

e. Date and time of reconstitution, nurse's initials

4.a. 1.5 g / 0.5 mL

b. 0.4 mL

c. No, the medication is only stable for 48 hours after reconstitution.

Worksheet: Multiple-Strength Reconstitution (p. 41 – 42)

1.a. All diluents can be used:
100 mL, 50 mL, or 20 mL

b. 100 mL of diluent added – give 75 mL
50 mL of diluent added – give 37.5 mL
20 mL of diluent added – give 15 mL

c. Date and time of reconstitution, nurse's initials, circle diluent amount and corresponding dosage strength.

2.a. 18.2 mL, 8.2 mL, or 3.2 mL

b. 18.2 mL of diluent added – 250,000 units / mL
8.2 mL of diluent added – 500,000 units / mL
3.2 mL of diluent added – 1,000,000 units / mL

c. 18.2 mL of diluent added – give 4 mL
8.2 mL of diluent added – give 2 mL
3.2 mL of diluent added – give 1 mL

d. The total amount of penicillin G potassium in the vial

3.a. 0.6 mL

b. The 2:00 AM dose will be the last full dose from the bottle. Only a partial dose (200,000 units) remains in the vial after the 2:00 AM dose is given.

c. The "Exp. 8/XX" is the date that the powdered medication (before reconstitution) loses its potency and will need to be discarded. This expiration date does not refer to the amount of time the mixed medication will remain stable.

4.a. Yes

b. 1420

Worksheet: Calculating mL / hr and Flow Rate (gtt / min) (p. 44)

1.a. 42 mL / hr
  b. 11 gtt / min

2.a. 63 mL / hr
  b. 63 gtt / min

3.a. 167 mL / hr
  b. 42 gtt / min

4.a. 180 mL / hr
  b. 30 gtt / min

5.a. 100 mL / hr
  b. 100 gtt / min

6.a. 125 mL / hr
  b. 31 gtt / min

Worksheet: Calculating Infusion and Completion Times (p. 45)

1. Infusion time   3 hr
   Completion time   0100

2. Infusion time   8 hr 30 min
   Completion time   1230

3. Infusion time   7 hrs
   Completion time   1800

4. Infusion time   3 hrs
   Completion time   1900

5. Infusion time 6 hr 48 min
   Completion time   0448

Worksheet: Labeling IV Bags (p. 46)

1.
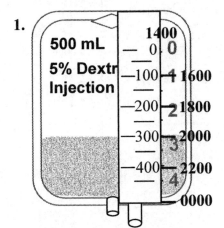

2.
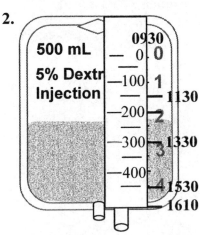

3.
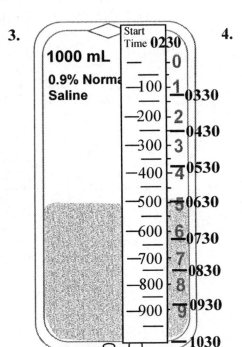

4.
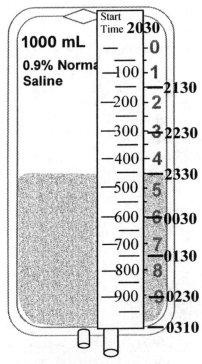

(Minutes worked to the hundredths place and rounded to a whole number).

(Minutes worked to the hundredths place and rounded to a whole number).

1. The nurse will take credit for 1200 mL on the PM shift.

2. The nurse will take credit for 650 mL on the night shift.
    The night shift nurse will give credit to the day shift for 350 mL of the primary IV.

3. The day shift nurse will take credit for 400 mL from the primary IV, and give credit to the
    day shift nurse for 325 mL at 1500.

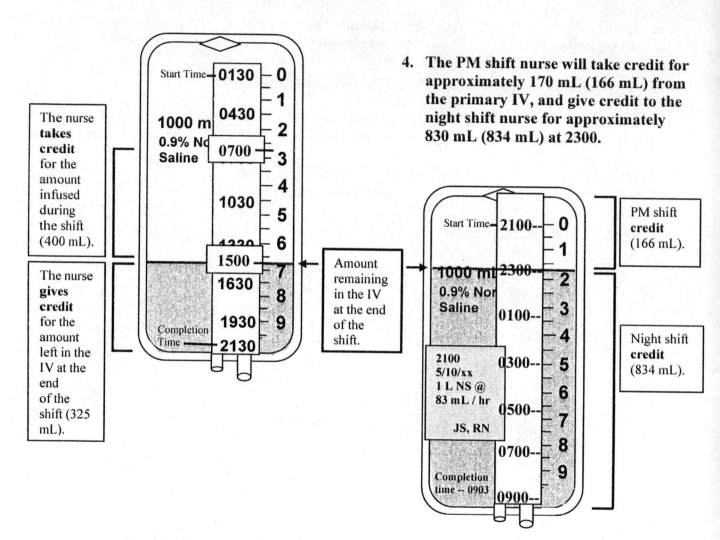

4. The PM shift nurse will take credit for
    approximately 170 mL (166 mL) from
    the primary IV, and give credit to the
    night shift nurse for approximately
    830 mL (834 mL) at 2300.

1. 3 min   2. 3 – 5 minutes   3. 2 minutes

Worksheet: **Administering Medications to Children (p. 50)**

1.

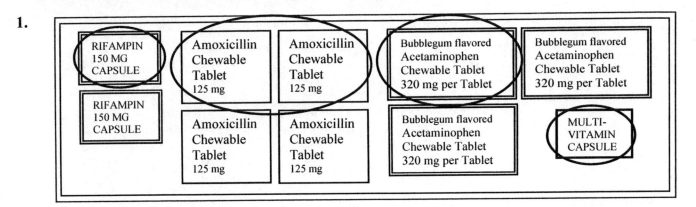

2. **Digoxin—a.** **KCl—b.** **Furosemide—b.**

Worksheet: Determining Safe Dose (p. 51)

1. Vincristine: Maximum safe dose: **1.48 mg**   Is ordered dose safe? **Yes**

    Asparaginase: Maximum safe dose: Is ordered dose safe? **Yes**
    20,000 International Units daily

    Prednisone: Maximum safe dose: **10 mg q.i.d.**   Is ordered dose safe? **No**

2. Cefuroxime: Maximum safe dose: **2 g q.12h.**   Is ordered dose safe? **Yes**

    Amikacin: Maximum safe dose: **200 mg q.8h.**   Is ordered dose safe? **Yes**

Worksheet: Nasogastric Fluid Replacement (p. 52)

1.a. **Maximum rate of replacement IV:**   **25 mL / hr**

    b. **Infusion Time of replacement IV:**   **2 hours 43 minutes**

    c. **Completion Time of replacement IV:**   **1713 or 5:13 PM**

2.a. **Maximum rate of replacement IV:**   **40 mL / hr**

    b. **Infusion Time of replacement IV:**   **3 hours 27 minutes**

    c. **Completion Time of replacement IV:**   **1942 or 7:42 PM**

Worksheet: Titration in Common Clinical Practice (p. 54 – 55)

1.   14 mL / hr

2.   10 mL / hr

3.   8 mg / hr

4.   Yes, the patient is receiving the correct dose.

5.   20 mL / hr

6.a. 60 mL / hr
  b. 80 mL / hr

7.   50 mL / hr

8.   9 mL / hr

Worksheet: Complex Titration Problems in Critical Care (p. 56 – 57)

1.a. 16.5 mg / hr – 33 mg / hr
  b. No, the infusion rate is too slow.
  c. 60 mg / hr – 240 mg / hr
  d. Yes, the IV is infusing at the lowest ordered rate.

2.a. 3 mL / hr
  b. 9 mL / hr

3.a. 47 mL / hr
  b. 108 mL / hr

4.   42 mL / hr

5.   125 mL / hr

Worksheet: Practice for the Licensure Exam (p. 59 – 62)

1. b. 20gtt /min

2. c. 2 0.3 mg sublingual tablets

3. a. 1 cup of coffee
    b. 6 ounces of apple juice
    d. 1/3 cup of orange-flavored gelatin
    e. a 90 mL lime popsicle

4. c. 1 cc insulin syringe with
        even and odd markings
    d. 1/2 cc insulin syringe

5.   17 mL / hr

6.   a 1 mL (tuberculin) syringe
        without a needle

7.

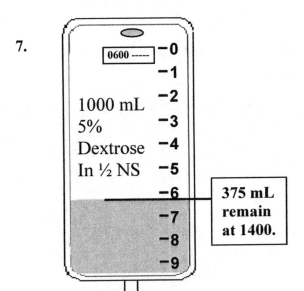

1000 mL 5% Dextrose In ½ NS

0600 -----

375 mL remain at 1400.

8.

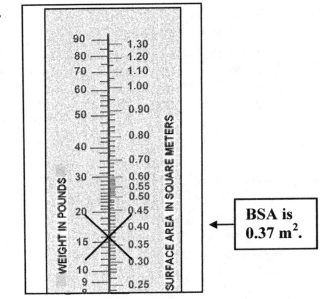

BSA is 0.37 m^2.

9. d. 21 units

10.   4 tablets

11.   **ORDERED OPTIONS**

Insert 1 mL air into the vial of diluent.

Withdraw 1 mL of diluent.

Insert diluent into the vial of powder.

Shake the vial.

Withdraw 1 mL of the mixed solution.

12.   c, d, b, a

Answers to Worksheets

Worksheet: Making Clinical Judgments in Medication Administration (p. 65–66)

1. a. **call the MD to clarify the order**

   CORRECT:

   The physician's order does not specify that the acetaminophen can be given for pain. A route of administration is not included. The order must be clarified before any acetaminophen can be given to the patient.

   INCORRECT:

   b. **administer two 325 mg tabs of acetaminophen.**
   The physician ordered the acetaminophen for fever, so the nurse cannot give the medication for joint pain without a change of order from the physician.

   c. **call the pharmacist.**
   The pharmacist could tell the nurse the routes available for acetaminophen, but the nurse can easily find out this information from a drug reference book.

2. b. **is incorrect, and requires further action because . . .**

   CORRECT:

   The purpose of an extended-release tablet is to release medication slowly over time. An extended-release tablet should never be crushed. Crushing (or chewing) extended-release or enteric-coated potassium tablets can cause GI irritation or ulceration of the gastric mucosa. As a High Alert drug, another concern is that the crushed potassium may have a faster than ordered absorption. The nurse should request that the pharmacist send a liquid form of potassium that can be administered through the NG tube.

   INCORRECT:

   a. **correctly follows the MD orders because . . .**
   The action of the nurse is not correct because of the reasons stated above. The physician needs to be called to report the error, and an incident report needs to be completed.

3. b. no, because . . .

CORRECT:

The total amount of insulin to be administered to the patient is correct. However, Nurse A needs to draw up each insulin dose in the presence of Nurse B, showing the insulin syringe with the needle still in the insulin bottle to Nurse B. Just showing the total amount of insulin in the syringe is not a safe check of these High Alert medications.

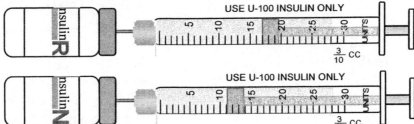

INCORRECT:

a. yes, because . . .

The action of the nurse is not correct because of the reasons stated above. The nurse should draw up the insulin again and follow the guidelines for the safe checking of insulin doses.

---

4. c. IV morphine sulfate and PO ibuprofen

CORRECT:

Ibuprofen 400 mg p.o. is ordered as an around-the-clock (ATC) medication. It is due at 1600, and should be given regardless of whether or not the patient receives a PRN dose of morphine sulfate.

Morphine sulfate 5 mg IV is ordered as needed for severe pain. The patient's self-report of pain is 8/10, so the patient needs to receive morphine sulfate as well as the ibuprofen. The last dose of morphine sulfate was at 1210, so the next dose can be given at 1610.

INCORRECT:

a. IV morphine sulfate

The patient's self-report of pain is 8/10, so the patient needs to receive morphine sulfate, as well as the around-the-clock scheduled dose of ibuprofen.

b. PO ibuprofen

The oral dose of ibuprofen will not adequately relieve the patient's severe pain. Therefore, both the ibuprofen and the morphine sulfate should be administered.

---

5. a. yes, because . . .

CORRECT:

The dosage strength of the amoxicillin suspension is 400 mg / 5 mL. 2 g (2000 mg) is contained in 25 mL. The nurse correctly reads the medicine cup at the bottom of the meniscus.

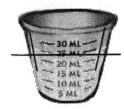

INCORRECT:

b. no, because . . .

The ordered dosage is contained in 25 mL. To read the medicine cup accurately, the nurse must read the bottom of the curved upper surface of the liquid (the meniscus).

1. c. correct, because . . .
CORRECT:

The directions for direct IV from the drug reference book state "each 1mg (10mL) of 1:10,000 solution [can be given] over at least 1 min". There are no specific instructions about the rate of administration for doses given over less than 1 minute. The safest course of action is to administer 1 mg (10 mL) <u>or any amount less than this</u> over at least 1 minute.

INCORRECT:
a. too rapid, because . . .
Rule of thumb: When there are no specific instructions about the rate of administration for doses smaller than those stated in the drug reference book, the safest action is to administer the drug over the amount of time specified in the drug book for a larger dose of the drug.
b. too slow, because . . .
The drug reference book gives no specific instructions about the rate of administration for a smaller dose of medication. It is unsafe to assume that a faster rate of administration is safe. Epinephrine is a High Alert drug. It is available in a variety of strengths, and it is essential that the nurse check the concentration of the drug very carefully. Patient harm or death may result from using a higher than ordered concentration or more rapid administration rate.

2. b. correctly set the rate of the blood infusion
CORRECT:

Each unit of PRBCs contains 250 mL. Two units (500 mL) is to infuse over 5 hours. To run the blood infusion at 100 mL / hour with a blood tubing of 10 gtt / mL, the nurse is correct to set the flow rate at 17 gtt / minute.

$$\frac{100\ mL\ /\ hr\ \ x\ 10\ gtt\ /\ mL}{60\ min} = 16.666\ or\ 17\ gtt\ /\ min$$

INCORRECT:
b.   made an error in setting the rate of the blood infusion.
The nurse correctly set the rate to infuse the two units of packed cells over 5 hours.

3. b. no, because . . .
CORRECT:
The nurse is correct to relabel the IV bag when there is a lapse of time between when an IV stops and when it can be restarted.
However, there are several errors in the relabeling of this IV:
- *The start time of the 1 liter of IV fluid (1700) is no longer on the IV label.*
- *The time the IV fluid was restarted (2000) should be at the level of the remaining IV fluid (between the numbers 1 and 2 on the IV bag). There are 850 mL remaining at 2000.*
- *The completion time of the liter of IV fluid (0600) is not labeled.*

INCORRECT:
a. yes, because . . .
The three components of labeling a flowmeter on an IV bag: start time, hourly intervals, and completion time of the IV, must be on every IV flow meter. There are several errors on this flowmeter.

4. c. too rapidly . . .
CORRECT:
The concentration of heparin in the IV is 100 units per mL. In order to infuse the IV heparin at 900 units / hour, the IV must run at 9 mL / hour. The setting on the IV pump is too rapid. Heparin is a High Alert medication. An overdose of heparin can cause bleeding. An attempt should be made to determine how long the patient has been receiving the incorrect dose of heparin. The physician should be notified, and follow-up coagulation lab studies (aPTT) are appropriate.

INCORRECT:
a. at the correct rate . . .
The IV is infusing too rapidly. Because heparin is a High Alert medication and a potent anticoagulant, the infusion rate should be double checked by another RN. In addition, the nurse should check the patient for any signs of bruising, bleeding, or hemmorhage.
b. too slowly . . .
The IV is infusing too rapidly. Recheck the titration calculation. The nurse should set the IV at 9 mL / hr, and notify the physician.

5. a. yes
CORRECT:
The nurse has recorded the correct amount of IV intake (950 mL) on the day shift I & O record. The day shift is from 0700 to 1500.

Primary IV:
　　375 mL of IV from 0700 to 1000 (3 hours @ 125 mL / hr.)
　　+375 mL of IV from 1000 to 1500 (5 hours @ 75 mL / hr.)
　　750 mL total for the shift

Secondary IVs:
　　100 mL from the vancomycin IVPB (given once in an 8-hour shift)
　　+100 mL from the pantoprazole IVPB (given @ 1100 on the day shift)
　　200 mL total for the shift

Total amount of IV intake (primary IV + secondary IVs):
　　750 mL
　　+200 mL
　　950 mL

INCORRECT:
b. no
The nurse has correctly entered the patient's intake and output on the I & O record.

Problem	Point Value	Answer
1.	(4 points)	18,207
2.	(4 points)	3682.29
3.	(4 points)	4054.0853
4.	(4 points)	20 2/9 or 20.22
5.	(4 points)	11 11/30 or 11.37
6.	(4 points)	24,468
7.	(4 points)	3.176
8.	(4 points)	40.318
9.	(4 points)	6 31/40 or 6.78
10.	(4 points)	2 19/20 or 2.95
11.	(4 points)	1,523,312
12.	(4 points)	2 1/7 or 2.14
13.	(4 points)	6 1/9 or 6.11
14.	(4 points)	127
15.	(4 points)	36.75525
16.	(4 points)	37.67
17.	(4 points)	0.4
18.	(4 points)	315
19.	(4 points)	2 5/6 or 2.83
20.	(4 points)	11/15 or 0.73
21.	(2 points)	XXVI
22.	(2 points)	XLVII
23.	(2 points)	XC
24.	(2 points)	LXXV
25.	(2 points)	XXXIX
26.	(2 points)	54
27.	(2 points)	2000
28.	(2 points)	13
29.	(2 points)	5 1/2
30.	(2 points)	84

Answers

Problem	Point Value	Answer
1.	(1 point)	Trade name: Diflucan
	(1 point)	Generic name: fluconazole
	(1 point)	Dosage strength: 10 mg / mL
	(1 point)	Give: 1 tsp
2.	(4 points)	149.6 lb
3.	(4 points)	2 tablets
4.	(2 points)	0.8 mL
	(2 points)	Shade in the prefilled cartridge:

5.	(1 point)	I – 860 mL
	(1 point)	O – 675 mL
	(1 point)	IV credit 500 mL
	(1 point)	Flow rate 125 gtt / min
6.	(4 points)	1.5 mL
7.	(2 points)	2.8 mL
	(2 points)	Shade in the syringe:

8.	(4 points)	Flow rate 32 gtt / min
9.	(1 point)	Safe loading dose: 319.6 mg
	(1 point)	Yes, the ordered loading dose is safe.
	(1 point)	Safe maintenance dose: 26.52 mg / hr for the 1st 12 hr, then 5.44 mg / hr to 10.88 mg / hr
	(1 point)	No, the ordered maintenance dose is not safe.
10.	(4 points)	720 mL
11.	(2 points)	Infusion time: 7 hrs 15 min
	(2 points)	Completion time: 0345 the next day

12. (2 points) 0.3 mL

(2 points) Shade in the most appropriate syringe:

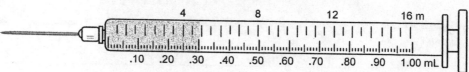

13. (4 points) 1.1 mL

14. (1 point) I -- 946 mL

(1 point) O -- 960 mL

(1 point) Amount remaining in the fat emulsion: 290 mL

(1 point) Amount remaining in the TPN: 400 mL

15. (2 points) 83 mL / hr

(2 points) 17 gtt / min

16. (1 point) Amount of diluent: 5 mL

(1 point) Type of diluent: 0.9% Sodium Chloride injection (without preservatives)

(1 point) Dosage strength: 38 mg / mL

(1 point) Give: 5.26 mL

17. (2 points) 4 hrs 30 minutes

(2 points) 2030 or 8:30 PM

18. (4 points) Flowmeter:

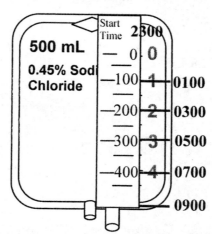

19. (2 points) Yes, the ordered dose is safe.

(2 points) No, the IV pump should be set at 120 mL / hr.

20. (4 points) 1.5 mL

21.   (1 point)   **Completion time: 0030**
        (2 points)   **Label the IV bag:**
        (1 point)   **Shade in IV bag:**

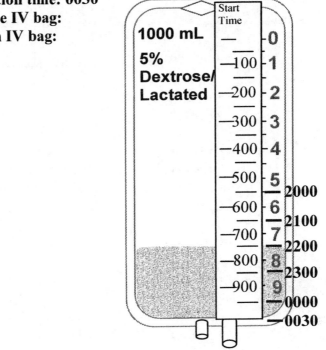

22.   (2 points)   **0.67 mL**
        (2 points)   **IV rate of administration: 3 – 5 minutes**

23.   (2 points)   **Maximum dose: 33 mg**
        (2 points)   **No, the ordered dose is too large.**

24.   (2 points)   **33 units**
        (2 points)   **Shade in the syringe:**

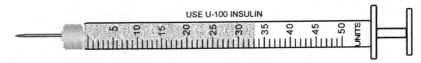

25.   (4 points)   **10 mL**

Answers

Problem	Point Value	Answer
1.	(2 points)	I — 1420 mL
	(2 points)	O — 625 mL
2.	(1 point)	Total amount in vial: 2 mL
	(1 point)	Controlled substance: Yes, Schedule II drug
	(1 point)	Dosage strength: 1000 mcg / 2 mL or 500 mcg / mL
	(1 point)	Give: 2 mL
3.	(4 points)	80 kg
4.	(4 points)	25 gtt / min
5.	(1 point)	Safe loading dose: 4.25 mg
	(1 point)	Yes, the ordered loading dose is safe.
	(1 point)	Safe infusion rate: 8.5 mg / hr
	(1 point)	No, the ordered infusion rate is not safe.
6.	(4 points)	79 mL
7.	(2 points)	Infusion time: 16 hrs 40 min
	(2 points)	Completion time: 0940 the next day
8.	(1 point)	Heparin 10,000 units / mL is most appropriate.
	(2 points)	Give 0.75 mL
	(1 point)	Shade in the syringe:

Problem	Point Value	Answer
9.	(1 point)	I -- 966 mL
	(1 point)	O -- 915 mL
	(1 point)	Amount remaining in the primary IV: 370 mL
	(1 point)	Amount remaining in the TPN: 114 mL
10.	(4 points)	42 mL / hr
11.	(1 point)	ankle: 3 cm
	(1 point)	lateral calf: 2.54 cm
	(1 point)	posterior calf: 25 cm
	(1 point)	hip: 3.25 cm

12.　　(2 points)　　**Infusion time: 7 hours 12 minutes**
　　　　　　(2 points)　　**Completion time: 1442 or 2:42 PM**

13.　　(4 points)　　**28 gtt / min**

14.　　(4 points)　　**Flowmeter:**

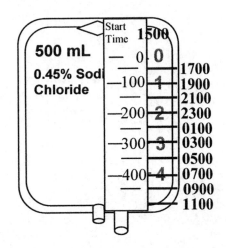

15.　　(2 points)　　**Amt. of diluent:**　　75 mL　33 mL　11.5 mL
　　　　　　(2 points)　　**Administer:**　　　44 mL　22 mL　11 mL

16.　　(4 points)　　**2 inches**

17.　　(4 points)　　**10 mL**
　　　　　　(2 points)　　**Shade in medicine cup:**

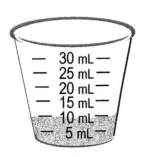

18.　　(2 points)　　**1.4 mL**
　　　　　　(2 points)　　**Shade in the most appropriate syringe:**

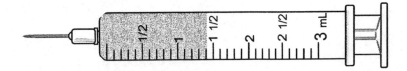

19.　　(2 points)　　**Administer: 18 mL**
　　　　　　(2 points)　　**IV rate of administration: 8 – 10 minutes**

20. (2 points)   Completion time: 2300

       (2 points)   Label the IV bag:

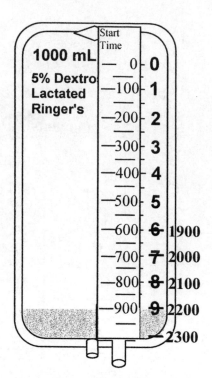

21. (2 points)   19 units

       (2 points)   Shade in the syringe:

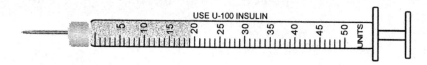

22. (2 points)   650 mL infused

       (2 points)   225 mL remain in the IV bag at 1500.

23. (2 points)   2.6 mg

       (2 points)   Yes, the ordered dose is safe.

24. (2 points)   1.5 mL

       (2 points)   Shade in the syringe:

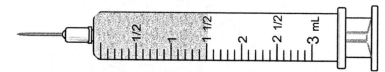

25. (2 points)   Yes, the ordered dose is safe.

       (2 points)   No, the IV rate should be 10 mL / hr.

Module: BASIC MATH REVIEW
Answers to Module Test I and II

Module Test I

1. 6074.6132

2. 87.755

3. 321.0155

4. 0.051

5. 1390.5

6. 0.001508

7. 45

8. 138.17

9. 736.78

10. 11/15 or 0.733

11. 6 1/2 or 6.5

12. 2 1/8 or 2.125

13. 9/20 or 0.45

14. 2 1/49 or 2.02

15. 2/225 or 0.009

16. 2

17. 59

18. 1999

19. 2

20. 28

Module Test II

1. 449.045

2. 553.75

3. 94.9922

4. 0.212

5. 2380

6. 0.000098

7. 1.4

8. 0.02

9. 1427.8

10. 17/21 or 0.809

11. 2 7/8 or 2.875

12. 5 1/6 or 5.167

13. 12/5, 2 2/5 or 2.4

14. 19 2/3 or 19.667

15. 1/75 or 0.013

16. 2 7/16 or 2.438

17. 44

18. 909

19. 11

20. 48

Module Test I

1. 3 ½ pills
2. 1 2/5 ounces or 1.4 ounces
3. 3 caplets
4. 2 tablets
5. 3 mL
6. 3 tablets
7. 2 tablets
8. 0.25 ounce or ¼ ounce
9. 2 tablets
10. 2.5 mL
11. 1.75 ounces or 1 ¾ ounces
12. 2 mL
13. 4 caplets
14. 1/2 tablet
15. 1.5 mL
16. 2 tablets
17. 4 mL
18. 0.75 mL
19. 4 tablets
20. 1.25 mL

Module Test II

1. 2 ½ tablets
2. 4 mL
3. 10 tablets
4. ½ tablet
5. 15 mL
6. 6 mL
7. 12 mL
8. 4 mL
9. 0.5 tablet
10. 11.25 mL
11. 5 mL
12. 2 mL
13. 2 tablets
14. 4 tablets
15. 2.5 mL
16. ¾ pill
17. 12.5 mL
18. 0.4 mL
19. 4 capsules
20. 2.5 mL

Answers to Module Test I and II

Module Test I

1. 0.025 km

2. 100 mg

3. 0.02 dL

4. 0.45 mg

5. 10,000 meters

6. 30 mL

7. 3 cm

8. 145.2 lb

9. 1 mL

10. 2 tablets

11. 0.5 mL

12. 2 mL

13. 3 tablets

14. 1/2 ounce

15. 3 tsp

16. 10 mL

17. 1 mL

18. 0.5 mL

19. 2 tablets

20. 0.75 mL

Module Test II

1. 500 mcg

2. ½ ounce

3. 6 tsp

4. 1 mL

5. 7.62 cm

6. 60 mL

7. 480 mL

8. 100 kg

9. 30 mL

10. 1 tablet

11. 1 mL

12. 4 mL

13. 2 tablets

14. 0.5 mL

15. 9.6 minims

16. 1.8 mL

17. 25 mL

18. 0.2 mL

19. 3 tablets

20. 0.25 mL

Module Test I

1. 745 mL
2. 940 mL
3. 600 mL
4. 650 mL
5. 814 mL
6. 500 mL
7. 550 mL
8. 650 mL
9. 375 mL
10. 725 mL
11. 775 mL
12. 125 mL
13. 250 mL
14. 100 mL
15. 80 mL
16. 237 mL
17. 119 mL
18. 711 mL
19. 100 mL
20. 500 mL

Module Test II

1. 1220 mL
2. 640 mL
3. 565 mL
4. 700 mL
5. 800 mL
6. 340 mL
7. 632 mL
8. 850 mL
9. 750 mL
10. 775 mL
11. 700 mL
12. 290 mL
13. 400 mL
14. 250 mL
15. 585 mL
16. 350 mL
17. 120 mL
18. 470 mL
19. 237 mL
20. 83 mL

Module: READING MEDICATION LABELS
Answers to Module Test I and II

Module Test I

1. Diflucan

2. 200 mg / tablet

3. p.o. or oral

4. 10,000 units / mL

5. 1 mL

6. multidose

7. Cortef

8. hydrocortisone

9. tablets

10. 20 mg / tablet

11. IM or IV

12. mL or liquid

13. 20 mg / 2 mL or 10 mg / mL

14. parenteral

15. multidose

16. true

17. true

18. true

19. true

20. false

Module Test II

1. Paxil

2. 20 mg / tablet

3. p.o. or oral

4. 1000 mcg / mL

5. 1 mL

6. multidose

7. Diflucan

8. fluconazole

9. tablets

10. 100 mg / tablet

11. IM or IV

12. mL or liquid

13. 100 mg / 2 mL or 50 mg / mL

14. parenteral

15. 2 mL

16. false

17. true

18. true

19. true

20. true

Module Test I

1. route of administration

2. frequency of administration

3. name of the drug

4. dose of the drug

5. route of administration

6. true

7. false; b.i.d. = 2x/day

8. false; frequency missing

9. false; names different

10. true

11. 1 capsule

12. 2 tablets

13. 2 tablets

14. 9 mL

15. 15 mL

16. 3 mL

17. 10 mL

18. 10 mL

19. 0.4 mL

20. 2 tablets

Module Test II

1. dose of the drug

2. route of administration

3. frequency of admin.

4. name of the drug

5. route of administration

6. true

7. true

8. false; q.i.d. = 4x/day

9. false; t.i.d. + bedtime = 4x/day

10. false; bedtime varies

11. 3 tablets

12. 1 tablet

13. 2 tablets

14. 0.75 mL

15. 10 mL

16. 30 mL

17. 5 mL

18. 10 mL

19. 10 mL

20. 1 capsule

Module Test I

1. B

2. D

3. D

4. D

5. B

6. A

7. D; change needle before administering

8. C

9. D

10. D

11. 3 mL 18G 1"

12. ½ cc 28G ½" insulin or 3/10 cc 31G 5/16" insulin

13. 2 mL 22G 1 ½" prefilled

14. 1 mL 25G 3/8"

15. 3 mL 25G 5/8"

16. 1 mL 25G 5/8"

17. 3 mL 22G 1 ½"

18. 1 mL 22G 1 ½"

19. ½ cc insulin

20. 1 mL 25G 5/8"

Module Test II

1. A

2. A

3. D

4. C

5. B

6. C

7. A

8. C

9. D

10. D

11. 3 mL 18G 1"

12. ½ cc 28G ½" insulin or 3/10 cc 28G ½" insulin

13. 2 mL 22G 1 ½" prefilled

14. 1 mL 25G 3/8"

15. 3 mL 25G 5/8"

16. 3 mL 22G 1 ½"

17. 3 mL 23G 1 ½"

18. 3 mL 22G 1 ½"

19. 1 cc insulin

20. 2 mL 25G 5/8" prefilled

Module Test I

1. 1 mL
2. 0.45 mL
3. 1.5 mL
4. 3 mL
5. 1.5 mL
6. 1.4 mL
7. 3.6 mL
8. 1.4 mL
9. 1.5 mL
10. 0.4 mL
11. 0.2 mL
12. 4 mL
13. 1 mL
14. 1.2 mL
15. 4 mL
16. 0.75 mL
17. 0.5 mL
18. 2 mL
19. 1.5 mL
20. 0.5 mL

Module Test II

1. 2.6 mL
2. 0.8 mL
3. 0.5 mL
4. 1 mL
5. 6 mL
6. 0.6 mL
7. 2.4 mL
8. 0.5 mL
9. 0.8 mL
10. 1.2 mL
11. 0.3 mL
12. 0.8 mL
13. 1 mL
14. 1.5 mL
15. 1 mL
16. 0.4 mL
17. 0.25 mL
18. 25 units
19. 22 units
20. 34 units

Module: RECONSTITUTION OF POWDERED MEDICATIONS
Answers to Module Test I and II

Module Test I

1. C
2. C
3. B
4. C
5. C
6. B
7. B
8. A
9. B
10. C
11. B
12. A
13. 2.1 mL
14. 12 mL
15. 1.25 mL
16. 3 mL
17. 4 mL
18. 0.25 mL
19. 0.3 mL
20. A

Module Test II

1. B
2. C
3. C
4. C
5. C
6. B
7. A
8. A
9. C
10. A
11. A
12. A
13. 0.6 mL
14. 20 mL
15. 0.75 mL
16. 2.7 mL
17. B
18. 1.8 mL
19. 3 mL
20. C

Module: IV CALCULATIONS
Answers to Module Test I and II

Module Test I

1. 63 ml / hr
2. 100 mL / hr
3. 50 gtt / min
4. 19 gtt / min
5. 6 minutes
6. 1 minute
7. 1 hour and 20 minutes
8. 4 hours and 48 minutes
9. 12 hours and 30 minutes
10. 6 hours and 40 minutes
11. 2140
12. 0930
13. 1515
14. 2210
15. 1330
16. 250 mL
17. 375 mL
18. 625 mL
19. 250 mL
20. 1840

Module Test II

1. 83 ml / hr
2. 83 ml / hr
3. 42 gtt / min
4. 25 gtt / min
5. 12 – 15 minutes
6. 2 minutes
7. 2 hours and 56 minutes
8. 6 hours and 12 minutes
9. 5 hours and 33 minutes
10. 6 hours and 27 minutes
11. 1800
12. 1340
13. 1720
14. 0840
15. 1130
16. 150 mL
17. 250 mL
18. 750 mL
19. 500 mL
20. 1815

Module Test I

1. 1.1 mg / dose

2. 50 mg / dose

3. 0.03 mg / day

4. Safe; max. dose = 316.67 mg

5. Not safe; max. dose = 332.5mg

6. Safe; max. dose = 100 mg

7. 10.8 mg / dose

8. 0.054 g / dose

9. 0.5 mg / dose

10. Not safe; max. dose = 4.65 mg

11. 7 hours

12. 3 hours

13. 1800

14. 2115

15. 909 mg / dose

16. 1 mg / dose

17. 5 – 10 mg / day

18. 475 – 760 mg b.i.d.

19. 1330

20. 0600

Module Test II

1. 0.136 mg / dose

2. 312.5 mg / dose

3. 435 mcg / day

4. Not safe; max. dose = 143.18 mg

5. Safe; max. dose = 583.33 mg

6. Safe; max. dose = 312.5 mg q.6h.

7. 1.35 mg / dose

8. 0.013 g / dose

9. 6.125 mg / dose

10. Not safe; max. dose = 9 mcg b.i.d.

11. 3 hours

12. 6 hours

13. 1950

14. 1220

15. 60 mg / day

16. 5.94 mg / dose

17. 187.5 – 375 mg q.6h.

18. 165 – 220 mg q.6 - 8 wks

19. 1557

20. 0017

Module Test I

1. 60 mL / hr
2. 35 mL / hr
3. 12 mL / hr
4. 30 mL / hr
5. 45 mL / hr
6. 20 mL / hr
7. 100 mL / hr
8. 1500 units / hr
9. 1000 units / hr
10. 8 mEq / hr
11. 75 mL / hr
12. 25 mL / hr
13. 25 mL / hr
14. 70 mL / hr
15. 48 mL / hr
16. 50 mL / hr
17. 45 mL / hr
18. 12 mL / hr
19. 40 mL / hr
20. 10 mL / hr

Module Test II

1. 25 mL / hr
2. 15 mL / hr
3. 9 mL / hr
4. 8 mL / hr
5. 6 mL / hr
6. 42 mL / hr
7. 20 mL / hr
8. 25 mEq / hr
9. 1300 units / hr
10. 8 mL / hr
11. 45 mL / hr
12. 16 mL / hr
13. 30 mL / hr
14. 30 mL / hr
15. 10 mL / hr
16. 12 mL / hr
17. 10 mL / hr
18. 45 mL / hr
19. 60 mL / hr
20. 60 mL / hr

In keeping with the NCLEX content of the CD and Student Workbook, the following answers provide rationales for both correct and incorrect responses.

Module Test 1

1. Option 4. 8 mL
Rationales:
1. Check the decimal point. The math is incorrect.
2. Check the decimal point. The math is incorrect.
3. The choice of 2 mg of morphine is incorrect. The patient's pain level of 8/10 requires that the nurse administer morphine sulfate 4 mg, not morphine sulfate 2 mg.
4. **The patient needs 4 mg of morphine sulfate for a pain level of 8/10. The correct dose to administer is 8 mL.**

2. Option 4. 890 mL
Rationales:
1. The math is incorrect. The intake from the IVPBs needs to be included in the parenteral intake.
2. The math is incorrect.
3. The math is incorrect. Two doses of the IVPB of metronidazole infused during the shift.
4. **Primary IV intake: 640 mL (primary IV @ 80 mL / hr for 8 hr) + 50 mL cefotaxime (1 dose in 8 hours) + 200 mL metronidazole (2 doses at 1600 and 2200) = 890 mL.**

3. Option 4. 1 ½ minutes
Rationales:
1. This IV push rate is too rapid.
2. This IV push rate is too rapid.
3. Each 100 mg needs to be given over at least 30 seconds, so 200 mg would take 60 seconds. The 50 additional mg also need to be given over the full amount of time: another 30 seconds, for a total of 90 seconds or 1 ½ minutes.
4. **Each 100 mg or fraction thereof needs to be given over at least 30 seconds.**

100 mg	--	30 seconds
100 mg	--	30 seconds
+ 50 mg	--	30 seconds
250 mg	--	90 seconds (or 1 ½ minute)

4. Option 4. c, b, a, d
Rationales:
1. The infusion time can only be calculated after step c and b.
2. Before the rate of the replacement IV can be calculated, the rate of the primary IV must be known.
3. Calculating the rate of the primary IV is the correct first step. Next, the rate of the replacement IV must be calculated.

4. The nurse first needs to know the rate of the primary IV (1 L q.8hr. = 125 mL / hr).
Subtracting the primary IV rate from the maximum hourly rate will provide the rate for
the IV replacement fluid (175 mL - 125 mL = 50 mL / hr).
Once the rate of the replacement IV is known, then the infusion time for the 250 mL can
be calculated. (5 hr). If the replacement IV starts at 12 midnight, the infusion time can
be added to 12 midnight to determine the completion time (12 AM + 5 hr = 5 AM).

5. **Option 1. 20 gtt / min**
Rationales:
1. **The formula for flow rate is $\frac{\text{mL x drop factor}}{\text{time in minutes}}$** $\frac{235 \text{ mL x 10 gtt / mL}}{2 \text{ hr x 60 min / hr}} = 20 \text{ gtt / min}$
2. This calculation is correct for unit # 2, not unit # 1.
3. The order is to infuse each unit over 2 hours. This answer is obtained if the flow rate for
unit # 1 is calculated over 1 hour.
4. The order is to infuse each unit over 2 hours. This answer is obtained if the flow rate for
unit # 2 is calculated over 1 hour.

6. **Option 2. IV intake for the day shift = 600 mL; 350 mL remain in the IV bag for the evening
shift.**
Rationales:
1. The IV contained only 950 mL at the start of the shift. The IV intake for the day shift is
incorrect. The amount remaining in the IV bag for the evening shift is correct.
2. **75 mL / hr for 8 hours = 600 mL (amount infused during the day shift).**
The IV contained 950 mL at 0700.
950 mL - 600 mL = 350 mL (amount remaining in the IV at 1500).
3. Both the IV intake and the amount remaining in the IV bag are incorrect. Look carefully at the
IV bag.
4. Both the IV intake and the amount remaining in the IV bag are incorrect. Look carefully at the
IV bag. Remember that the IV contained only 950 mL at the start of the shift.

7. **Option 2. The drug is powdered and needs to be reconstituted.**
Option 3. The drug is for parenteral administration only.
Rationales:
1. There is no dosage strength on the drug label. The 1 gram is the total amount of Ancef in the
vial. The dosage strength will be found with the mixing instructions on the package insert.
2. **The lack of a dosage strength on the drug label is a clue that this is a powdered drug that
must be reconstituted. The words "reconstituted Ancef" are present in small lettering
on the package label.**
3. **The drug is for IV or IM use only. Both of these are parenteral routes for medication
administration.**
4. There are no mixing instructions on the outside of the package. Instructions for reconstitution
can be found on the package insert.

8. **Option 2. 2 tablets**
Rationales:
1. The calculation is incorrect. 250 mg must be converted to grams (0.25 g). Check the setup
for the problem.

Module Test 1 (con't)

2. **250 mg = 0.25 g (ordered amount)**
   0.125 mg = amount in each tablet
   The ordered amount is contained in 2 tablets.
3. The calculation is incorrect. 3 tablets is more than the ordered dose.
4. The calculation is incorrect. 6 tablets is more than the ordered dose.

9. **Option 1. 0.25 mL**
   Rationales:
   1. **The Carpuject prefilled syringe contains a total amount of 1 mL of hydromorphone (dosage strength = 2 mg / mL). The remaining space (1 ½ mL) is empty. The nurse is to administer 1.5 mg, which is contained in 0.75 mL (amount to be administered).**
      1.00 mL (total amount in the Carpuject prefilled syringe
      - 0.75 mL (amount to be administered)
      0.25 mL (amount to be discarded)
   2. 0.75 mL is the amount to be administered, not the amount to be discarded.
   3. There is only 1 mL in the Carpuject prefilled syringe. The remaining space (1 ½ mL) is empty.
   4. There is only 1 mL in the Carpuject prefilled syringe. The remaining space (1 ½ mL) is empty.

10. **Option 2. with 4 units of Humulin R insulin in a ½ cc insulin syringe.**
    Rationales:
    1. A total of 39 units of insulin must be administered. A 3/10 cc insulin syringe only holds 30 units.
    2. **35 units of NPH insulin and 4 units of Humulin R insulin can be mixed in the same syringe. 35 + 4 = 39 units. This amount of insulin can best be measured in a ½ cc insulin syringe, which holds up to 50 units and can measure both even and odd numbers of units.**
    3. A total of 39 units of insulin must be administered. A 1 cc insulin syringe will only measure even numbers of units. 39 units is an odd number of units that cannot be measured accurately.
    4. NPH and Humulin R insulin can be mixed in the same syringe. There is no need to give the patient two injections of insulin.

Module Test 2

1. **Option 3. 0.4 mL of the 20,000 units / mL vial of heparin**
   Rationales:
   1. Check the decimal point. The correct answer using this strength of heparin is 8 mL.
   2. Although this answer is correct mathematically, 8 mL is too much to administer subcutaneously into the abdomen. The 20,000 units / mL vial is the better choice.
   3. **The 20,000 unit / mL vial of heparin is the correct choice. The correct answer using this vial of heparin is 0.4 mL.**
   4. Check the decimal point. The correct answer using this strength of heparin is 0.4 mL.

Module Test 2 (con't)

2. **Option 3. 18 mL / hr**
   Rationales:
   1. Check the decimal point. The correct answer is 18 mL / hr.
   2. The calculation is incorrect. Check the decimal point, and don't forget to use the patient's weight in the calculation.
   3. **The order is for 0.5 mcg / kg/ min. This patient weighs 60 kg.**
      0.5 mcg / kg / min x 60 kg = 30 mcg / min
      30 mcg / min x 60 min = 1800 mcg / hour
      1800 mcg / hr = 1.8 mg / hour
      Applying the formula, the answer is 18 mL / hr
   4. The calculation is incorrect. Don't forget to use the patient's weight in the calculation.

3. **Option 1. 75 mL**
   Option 2. 33 mL
   Option 4. 11.5 mL
   Rationales:
   1. **The reconstitution instructions give the nurse 3 choices for the amount of diluent. 75 mL is correct.**
   2. **The reconstitution instructions give the nurse 3 choices for the amount of diluent. 33 mL is correct.**
   3. The reconstitution instructions must be followed exactly. 23 mL is not listed as an amount of diluent to add, therefore this amount of diluent cannot be used. It is not correct to double or change any diluent amount.
   4. **The reconstitution instructions give the nurse 3 choices for the amount of diluent. 11.5 mL is correct.**

4. **Option 4. The maximum dose is 500 mg. The ordered dose is not safe.**
   Rationales:
   1. The calculation of the maximum dose is not correct.
   2. The calculation of the maximum dose is not correct. Remember to change the patient's weight to kilograms.
   3. It is not correct to use 33.3 mg / kg / q.8h. to calculate this dose, because the order is for a medication that is to be administered q.6h. It is most accurate to compare the physician's order with the maximum dose in the drug reference book with the same time interval between doses (q.6h.).
   4. **The patient weighs 44 lbs = 20 kg. The ordered medication is to be given q.6h.**
      It is most accurate to compare the ordered dose with the maximum dose recommended in the drug reference book q.6h. (25 mg / kg). 600 mg is ordered; 500 mg is the maximum recommended dose. The ordered dose is too much, and therefore is not safe. The nurse should call the doctor to clarify the order.

5. **Option 1. "1 tsp every 4 hours when my son coughs."**
   Option 2. "5 mL in the medicine spoon as needed every four hours."
   Rationales:
   1. **100 mg of guaifenesin is ordered. 100 mg is contained in 5 mL. 5 mL = 1 tsp.**
   2. **100 mg of guaifenesin is ordered. 100 mg is contained in 5 mL.**

Module Test 2 (con't)

3. The child is to receive 5 mL every 4 hours as needed. A tablespoon = 15 mL and ½ tablespoon = 7.5 mL, which is more than the doctor ordered.
4. The child is to receive 5 mL every 4 hours as needed. 5 mL = 1 teaspoon, not 1 tablespoon.

6. Option 3. 1.6 mL
Rationales:
1. Check the decimal point. The calculation is incorrect.
2. The calculation is incorrect.
3. **The label on the prefilled syringe of fentanyl contains 3 different dosage strengths. Any of them can be used. The answer to the calculation is 1.6 mL.**
4. The calculation is incorrect.

7. Option 2. 21 gtt / min
Rationales:
1. The calculation is incorrect.
2. **The formula for flow rate is** $\underline{\text{mL x drop factor}}$ $\qquad \dfrac{1000 \text{ mL x } 15 \text{ gtt / mL}}{12 \text{ hr x } 60 \text{ min / hr}} = 21 \text{ gtt / min}$
   $\qquad\qquad\qquad\qquad\quad$ time in minutes
3. The IV will infuse at 83 mL / hr, not 83 gtt / min.
4. The calculation is incorrect.

8. Option 1. calculate if the ordered dose is a safe dose for this patient.
Option 3. identify the dosage strength of the prepared solution.
Option 4. use a drug reference book to find the recommended rate of administration.
Rationales:
1. **The nurse must check to see that the ordered dose is a safe dose for this patient.**
2. There is no need to call the pharmacist as this information is available on the drug label.
3. **The dosage strength of the prepared solution is needed to calculate the amount to give to the patient.**
4. **The rate of administration for each IV medication must be researched. This information is available in a drug reference book.**

9. Option 2. Intake 1485 mL / Output 750 mL
Rationales:
1. The intake is incorrect. Remember to add the IVPB to the parenteral intake. The output is also incorrect. The wound drainage needs to be included in the output.
2. **Parenteral intake –**

Primary IV: 0700 to 1000: (125 mL / hr x 3 hr = 375 mL)	**375 mL**	
1100 to 1500: (125 mL / hr x 4 hr = 500 mL)	**500 mL**	
IVPB (ceftazidime): 1200:	**+ 50 mL**	
Total IV intake:	**925 mL**	

Oral intake: (water)	50 mL
(1 cup ice chips)	120 mL
(4 oz milk)	120 mL
(6 oz broth)	180 mL
(3 oz JELL-O)	+ 90 mL
	560 mL

Module Test 2 (con't)

Total intake: 925 mL + 560 mL = 1485 mL

Total output: (urinary catheter)   450 mL
(voided urine)   250 mL
(wound drain)   + 50 mL
           750 mL

3. The intake is incorrect. The IV infiltrated and did not infuse for 1 hour during the shift. The output is correctly calculated.
4. The intake is incorrect. Remember that ice melts to ½ of its volume. The output is incorrect Remember to record the voided urine as output.

10. Option 3. 200 mL
Rationales:
1. 950 mL was in the bag at the start of the shift, not at 1500.
2. The IV rate was increased for 2 hours. 350 mL would have been left if the IV infused at 75 mL / hr for the entire shift.
3. **The total amount of IV infused for the shift is 750 mL –**

0700 to 1000 --	225 mL
1000 to 1200 --	300 mL
+ 1200 to 1500 --	225 mL
Total --	750 mL

Starting amount --	950 mL
	- 750 mL
	200 mL

4. Recheck the calculation. This answer is incorrect.

Module Test 3

1. Option 3. 0.86 m^2
Rationales:
1. If a line is drawn between 50 lbs and 45 inches, the BSA is 0.86 m^2. To obtain this answer, 45 cm was used, not 45 inches.
2. If a line is drawn between 50 lbs and 45 inches, the BSA is 0.86 m^2. To obtain this answer, 50 kg and 45 cm were used, not 50 lbs and 45 inches.
3. **If a line is drawn between 50 lbs and 45 inches, the BSA is 0.86 m^2.**
4. If a line is drawn between 50 lbs and 45 inches, the BSA is 0.86 m^2. To obtain this answer, 50 kg was used, not 50 lbs.

2. Option 2. 1.9 mL
Rationales:
1. After reconstitution, the dosage strength of the levothyroxine is 40 mcg / mL. 200 mcg is the total amount of levothyroxine in the vial. This number should not be used in the calculation.
2. **After reconstitution, the dosage strength of the levothyroxine is 40 mcg / mL. The order is for 0.075 mg (75 mcg). The nurse will administer 1.875 mL (or 1.9 mL).**

3. The dosage strength that should be used in the calculation is 40 mcg / mL. Check the decimal point in the calculation.
4. The correct amount to administer is 1.875 mL or 1.9 mL. Check the decimal point.

3. Option 2. 25 gtt / min
  Rationales:
  1. This flow rate is not correct. The drop factor (15 gtt / mL) must be used in the calculation.

  2. **Using the formula $\dfrac{\text{\# mL x drop factor}}{\text{time in minutes}}$:   the flow rate is 25 gtt / min.**

  3. Flow rate is measured in gtt / min. The drop factor (15 gtt / mL) must be used in the calculation.
  4. Flow rate is measured in gtt / min. The calculation is correct, but the answer is not labeled correctly.

4. Option 1. Zofran is the trade name of the medication.
  Option 4. The patient should be directed to take 1 tablet two times a day.
  Rationales:
  1. **Zofran is the trade name of the medication. Notice the registered trademark symbol after the name Zofran.**
  2. Read the small print on the label carefully. The dosage strength of the medication is 4 mg / tablet.
  3. The bottle of medication contains 30 tablets. If the patient takes 4 mg (1 tablet) twice a day, the bottle will last for only 15 days.
  4. **Each tablet contains 4 mg of ondansetron hydrochloride. The patient is to take 4 mg twice a day. The directions are correct.**

5. Option 2. Intake 550 mL / Output 275 mL
  Rationales:
  1. The intake includes the primary IV and the IVPB. Don't forget the intake for the hour that the IV was infusing after it was restarted. The intake = 500 mL from the primary IV, plus 50 mL from the IVPB = 550 mL.
  The urine output is correctly calculated.
  2. **Intake: The IV of LR infused at 125 mL / hr for 4 hours**
           (1800 – 2100 = 3 hours; 2200 – 2300 = 1 hr).
           125 mL / hr x 4 hr = 500 mL.
           The patient also received an IVPB with 50 mL D5W.
           500 mL + 50 mL = 550 mL.
     Urine output: Calculate the true urine output by subtracting the amount of irrigant that
                 infused into the bladder (500 mL between 1800 and 2300) from the total
                 amount in the urinary drainage bag (775 mL).
                 775 - 500 = 275 mL of urine.
  3. The calculation of the IV intake starts at 1800, not 1500. The IV infused for only 4 hours during the 1500 – 2300 shift, not for the full shift. The primary IV intake = 500 mL.
  Adding the 50 mL from the IVPB, the total intake is 550 mL.
  Not all of the fluid in the urinary drainage bag is urine. The true urine output is calculated by

subtracting the amount of irrigant that infused into the bladder (500 mL between 1800 and 2300) from the total amount in the urinary drainage bag (775 mL). 775 - 500 = 275 mL of urine.

4. The IV infused for 4 hours only during the 8-hour shift.
Not all of the fluid in the urinary drainage bag is urine. The true urine output is calculated by subtracting the amount of irrigant that infused into the bladder (500 mL) from the total amount in the urinary drainage bag (775 mL) = 275 mL of urine.

6. **Option 2. The IV pump should be set at 16 mL / hr at 1200. The IV pump should be set at 18 mL / hr at 1800.**

Rationales:

1. The IV pump setting for 1200 is correct; The APTT is not in the therapeutic range, so the standard heparin adjustment scale must be consulted. For an APTT value of 50 seconds and a patient weight of 50 kg, the IV pump is to be *increased* by 2 mL, not set at 2 mL.

2. **An IV with 25,000 units of heparin in 500 mL 0.45% NaCl has a concentration of 50 units / mL. To administer 800 units / hr, the IV pump must be set at 16 mL / hr. Since the APTT is not in the therapeutic range, the standard heparin adjustment scale (for the APTT value and patient's weight of 50 kg) states to increase the rate of the IV by 2 mL from the starting rate. 16 mL + 2 mL = 18 mL / hr.**

3. The rate of the IV pump at 1200 is not correct. The starting rate for the IV pump should be 16 mL / hr. Due to the low APTT value at 1800, the rate of the IV pump should be increased by 2 mL / hr, but because the starting rate was incorrect, the adjusted rate is also incorrect.

4. The rate of the IV pump at 1200 is not correct. The starting rate for the IV pump should be 16 mL / hr. Due to the low APTT value at 1800, the rate of the IV pump should be increased by 2 mL / hr, but because the starting rate was incorrect, the adjusted rate is also incorrect.

7. **Option 3. 79 mL**

Rationales:

1. 316 mL is the total amount of mixed solution (Nepro and water), not the amount of water to add.
2. 178 mL is not a correct answer. Recheck the math.
3. **79 mL added to a 237 mL can of Nepro makes a ¾-strength tube feeding solution.**
4. 59 mL is not a correct answer. Recheck the math.

8. **Option 2. 15.8 mg / hr is the maximum dose. The ordered dose is safe.**

Rationales:

1. 6 *mL* / hr is the maximum rate of the drug, not the maximum dose in mg. The conclusion is correct, but the work supporting the conclusion is not.

2. **The child weighs 20 kg (44 lb = 20 kg). The maintenance dose of aminophylline is 0.79 mg / kg x 20 kg = 15.8 mg / hr. The physician's order is less than 15.8 mg / hr, and is therefore a safe dose.**

3. The calculation is correct. The maximum safe dose of aminophylline is 15.8 mg / hr. The conclusion is incorrect: the physician's order is less than the maximum hourly dose, and is therefore safe.

4. The maximum safe rate must be calculated using the child's weight in kg, not lbs. The child weighs 44 lbs = 20 kg. The conclusion is not correct, and the work supporting the conclusion is also incorrect.

Module Test 3 (con't)

9. **Option 4. 2 mL**
   Rationales:
   1. The math is incorrect. Check the decimal point.
   2. The math is incorrect. The nurse should administer 2 mL.
   3. The math is incorrect. The nurse should administer 2 mL.
   4. **0.1 mg = 100 mcg. 100 mcg is contained in 2 mL.**

10. **Option 1. Yes, 7500 units are contained in 0.75 mL.**
    Rationales:
    1. **The dosage strength of the heparin is 10,000 units / 1 mL. 7500 units are contained in 0.75 mL. The tuberculin syringe can measure to the hundredths place accurately. The nurse has prepared the correct amount of heparin for the patient.**
    2. The tuberculin syringe is the most accurate syringe available in clinical practice. The dose is correct and the syringe has been correctly prepared with 7500 units of heparin.
    3. The amount drawn up in the syringe is correct.
    4. The amount drawn up in the syringe is correct.

Module Test 4

1. **Option 3. Flowmeter # 3**
   Rationales:
   1. This flowmeter lists the start time as 2200, instead of 2000. Therefore, the labeling of the IV flowmeter is incorrect. In addition, the flowmeter does not include a completion time.
   2. This flowmeter lists the start time of 2200 correctly, and the decreased rate begins at 2200. The military time as listed is incorrect. After 2400, the time for the next 125 mL should be 0100, not 2500. Military time runs from 0000 hours to 2400 hours.
   3. **This flowmeter is correctly labeled with the start time, hourly intake, and completion time of the IV fluid.**
   4. This flowmeter lists the start time as 2200, instead of 2000. The hourly rate on the IV flowmeter is labeled correctly. However, the flowmeter does not include a completion time.

2. **Option 2. Intake 1270 mL / Output 750 mL**
   Rationales:
   1. The patient's oral and parenteral intake includes: 6 oz broth = 180 mL, 4 ounce juice = 120 mL, 8 ounces of ice chips (ice chips melt to 1/2 the original amount, or 4 ounces) = 120 mL, 800 mL IV intake (100 mL / hr for 8 hours), and 50 mL IVPB at 0900.
       (180 mL + 120 mL + 120 mL + 800 mL + 50 mL = 1270 mL)
       The output includes emesis of 200 mL, and voided urine output of 225 mL and 325 mL.
       (200 mL + 225 mL + 325 mL = 750 mL)
   2. **The oral and parenteral intake and output have been correctly calculated.**
   3. The patient's oral and parenteral intake includes: 6 oz broth = 180 mL, 4 ounce juice = 120 mL, 8 ounces of ice chips (ice chips melt to 1/2 the original amount, or 4 ounces) = 120 mL, 800 mL IV intake (100 mL / hr for 8 hours), and 50 mL IVPB at 0900.
       (180 mL + 120 mL + 120 mL + 800 mL + 50 mL = 1270 mL)
       The output includes emesis of 200 mL, and voided urine output of 225 mL and 325 mL.
       (200 mL + 225 mL + 325 mL = 750 mL)

Module Test 4 (con't)

4. The patient's oral and parenteral intake includes: 6 oz broth = 180 mL, 4 ounce juice = 120 mL, 8 ounces of ice chips (ice chips melt to 1/2 the original amount, or 4 ounces) = 120 mL, 800 mL IV intake (100 mL / hr for 8 hours), and 50 mL IVPB at 0900.

    (180 mL + 120 mL + 120 mL + 800 mL + 50 mL = 1270 mL)

    The output includes emesis of 200 mL, and voided urine output of 225 mL and 325 mL.

    (200 mL + 225 mL + 325 mL = 750 mL)

3. **Option 1. 3/10 cc insulin syringe**
   Option 2. 1/2 cc insulin syringe
   Rationales:
   1. **The nurse needs to administer the 6 units of regular insulin and the 23 units of NPH together, for a total of 29 units. The 3/10 cc insulin syringe can accurately measure odd-numbered units of insulin.**
   2. **The nurse needs to administer the 6 units of regular insulin and the 23 units of NPH together, for a total of 29 units. The 1/2 cc insulin syringe can accurately measure odd-numbered units of insulin.**
   3. The nurse needs to administer the 6 units of regular insulin and the 23 units of NPH together, for a total of 29 units. The 1 cc insulin syringe cannot accurately measure odd-numbered units of insulin. The 1 cc insulin syringe is calibrated to measure even-numbered units accurately.
   4. The tuberculin syringe should not be used to measure insulin doses. Insulin syringes are calibrated to measure insulin accurately.

4. **Option 3. 2 mL**
   Rationales:
   1. Recheck the calculation. The dosage strength on the prefilled syringe is 0.25 mg / mL. The ordered amount is 0.5 mg.
   2. Recheck the calculation. The dosage strength on the prefilled syringe is 0.25 mg / mL. The ordered amount is 0.5 mg.
   3. **Based on the dosage strength of the prefilled syringe, 2 mL is the correct dose.**
   4. Recheck the calculation. The dosage strength on the prefilled syringe is 0.25 mg / mL. The ordered amount is 0.5 mg.

5. **Option 4. 5 mL**
   Rationales:
   1. After reconstitution, the resulting dosage strength is 40 mcg / mL. To administer the ordered dose accurately, the nurse must convert mg to mcg by moving the decimal point 3 places from left to right (0.20 mg = 200 mcg). The nurse will administer 5 mL.
   2. After reconstitution, the resulting dosage strength is 40 mcg / mL. To administer the ordered dose accurately, the nurse must convert mg to mcg by moving the decimal point 3 places from left to right (0.20 mg = 200 mcg). The nurse will administer 5 mL.
   3. After reconstitution, the resulting dosage strength is 40 mcg / mL. To administer the ordered dose accurately, the nurse must convert mg to mcg by moving the decimal point 3 places from left to right (0.20 mg = 200 mcg). The nurse will administer 5 mL.
   4. **After reconstitution, the resulting dosage strength is 40 mcg / mL. The problem has been calculated correctly.**

Module Test 4 (con't)

6. **Option 1. 5 min**
   Rationales:
   1. **After dilution, the recommended rate of administration for the ordered dose should be over 5 min.**
   2. The recommended rate of administration for the IV push medication is 5 min.
   3. The rate for direct IV should be used, not that for intermittent infusion. The recommended rate of administration is 5 min.
   4. The rate for direct IV should be used, not that for intermittent infusion. The recommended rate of administration is 5 min.

7. **Option 2. 400 mL**
   Rationales:
   1. The IV infused at 100 mL for 2 hours (0900 – 1100) = 200 mL. The rate was increased to 150 mL / hr for 2 hrs (1100 – 1300) = 300 mL. The IV infused at 100 mL / hr for 1 hr (1300 – 1400) = 100 mL. Total parenteral intake is 600 mL. 400 mL remains in the IV bag at 1400.
   2. **This is the correct amount left in the IV bag at 1400.**
   3. The IV infused at 100 mL for 2 hours (0900 – 1100) = 200 mL. The rate was increased to 150 mL / hr for 2 hrs (1100 – 1300) = 300 mL. The IV infused at 100 mL / hr for 1 hr (1300 – 1400) = 100 mL. Total parenteral intake is 600 mL. 400 mL remains in the IV bag at 1400.
   4. 600 mL is the amount that has infused into the patient. 400 mL is the amount that remains in the IV bag at 1400.

8. **Option 3. should not administer 1 mL of this drug at this time.**
   Option 4. cannot calculate the ordered dose based on the label information.
   Rationales:
   1. To administer the ordered dose safely, the nurse needs to know and follow the reconstitution instructions. The reconstitution instructions are not listed on the label. The nurse needs to look at the information found in the package insert to gather this information.
   2. The nurse needs to read the reconstitution information found in the package insert to identify the recommended solution for reconstitution.
   3. **The nurse needs to reconstitute the medication according to the manufacturer's recommendations. The reconstitution instructions are not on the drug label. The nurse should not administer the medication without following the reconstitution information.**
   4. **Based on the information from this drug label, the nurse does not have the appropriate information for reconstituting this medication.**

9. **Option 1. There is a potential for drug abuse leading to physical and psychological dependence.**
   Rationales:
   1. **The symbol, C-III, indicates the potential for drug abuse. Drugs labeled with a C-I, C-II, C-III, C-IV, and C-V are identified by the Drug Enforcement Agency (DEA) to have the potential for abuse and physical and psychological dependency.**
   2. The prefilled syringe contains 1 mL of Buprenorphine hydrochloride. 1.5 mL is empty.
   3. The medication may be given IV or IM only.
   4. The rate of administration is not known from the drug label. The nurse needs to research the rate of administration for this drug in a drug reference book

Module Test 4 (con't)

10. **Option 2. 24 gtt / min**
    Rationales:
    1. After calculating, the answer is 23.6 gtt / min. The nurse should apply the rounding rules and round the answer to 24 gtt / min.
    2. **The nurse has correctly calculated and rounded the answer for the whole blood infusion.**
    3. This flow rate would infuse the whole blood over 1 hour, not the ordered 3 hours.
    4. This flow rate would infuse the whole blood over 1 hour, not the ordered 3 hours.

Module Test 5

1. **Option 3. The next IV should be hung at 1830.**
    Rationales:
    1. The IV was started at 0730 and infused at 75 mL for 4 hours for a total intake of 300 mL. The IV rate was increased to 100 mL per hour starting at 1130. From 1130 to 1500, the parenteral intake was another 350 mL. The nurse administered 100 mL from the IVPB. The total parenteral intake was 750 mL for the shift.
    2. The 75 mL per hour rate was ordered for the first IV only. The IV fluid should infuse at 100 mL per hour.
    3. **The IV infused at 75 mL / hr for the first 4 hours, then the rate was increased to 100 mL / hr. At 1500, the IV had 350 mL remaining. The nurse is correct to anticipate that the IV bag will be completed in 3.5 hours or 1830.**
    4. The famotidine is ordered IVP.

2. **Option 2. correct estimated fluid level and correct time.**
    Rationales:
    1. The flowmeter is labeled with the correct estimated fluid level and time to monitor the ordered hourly rate of 75 mL / hr.
    2. **The flowmeter is labeled with the correct estimated fluid level and time to monitor the ordered hourly rate of 75 mL / hr.**
    3. The starting amount was 775 mL at 0900. The flowmeter is labeled with the correct estimated fluid level and time to monitor the ordered hourly rate of 75 mL / hr.
    4. The IV infused from 0700 to 0800, for another 75 mL of IV intake. The starting amount at 0900 was 775 mL. The flowmeter is labeled with the correct estimated fluid level and time to monitor the ordered hourly rate of 75 mL / hr.

3. **Option 1. 0.5 mL**
    Rationales:
    1. **The dosage strength of the alfentanil is 500 mcg / mL. Alfentanil 0.25 mg is ordered. 0.25 mg is equivalent to 250 mcg. After calculating, the nurse is correct to withdraw 0.5 mL into the syringe.**
    2. This calculation is incorrect. The ordered dose, 0.25 mg, is equivalent to 250 mcg. After calculating, the nurse will administer 0.5 mL.
    3. This calculation is incorrect. The ordered dose, 0.25 mg, is equivalent to 250 mcg. After calculating, the nurse will administer 0.5 mL.
    4. This calculation is incorrect. The ordered dose, 0.25 mg, is equivalent to 250 mcg. After calculating, the nurse will administer 0.5 mL.

Module Test 5 (con't)

4. **Option 4. 3 minutes**
   Rationales:
   1. The recommended rate of administration is 100 mcg over 1 min. The ordered dose is 0.3 mg, which is equivalent to 300 mcg. Administering 300 mcg over 30 seconds is too fast.
   2. The recommended rate of administration is 100 mcg over 1 min. The ordered dose is 0.3 mg, which is equivalent to 300 mcg. Administering 300 mcg over 1 minute is too fast.
   3. The recommended rate of administration is 100 mcg over 1 min. The ordered dose is 0.3 mg, which is equivalent to 300 mcg. Administering 300 mcg over 2 minutes is too fast.
   4. **The rate of administration for 300 mcg is:**

   > **100 mcg — 1 minute**
   > **100 mcg — 1 minute**
   > **+ 100 mcg — 1 minute**
   > **300 mcg — 3 minutes**

5. **Option 2. Reconstitute with 9.6 mL of 0.9% NaCl.**
   Option 3. Withdraw 5 mL of reconstituted solution.
   Rationales:
   1. The nurse has a 1 gram vial. The addition of 4.8 mL of D5W is to reconstitute the drug contained in the 500 mg vial.
   2. **This is the correct amount for reconstituting the drug contained in the 1 gram vial.**
   3. **The reconstituted solution yields a dosage strength of 100 mg / mL The order is to administer 500 mg of ceftriaxone.**
   4. The nurse must give the ordered amount based on the vial size and resulting dosage strength.

6. **Option 3. 270 mL**
   Rationales:
   1. To make a ¼-strength formula the nurse must add 270 mL of water.
   2. To make a ¼-strength formula the nurse must add 270 mL of water.
   3. **Adding 270 mL of water to the 90 mL of formula will make a ¼-strength formula solution.**
   4. Adding 360 mL of water to the 90 mL of formula will dilute the formula too much. 360 mL is the total amount of the mixed solution, not the amount of water to add.

7. **Option 2. The maximum dose is 167.99 mcg. The ordered dose is safe.**
   Rationales:
   1. 83.99 mcg is the minimum dose for a child who weighs 42 lbs. The nurse needs to calculate the maximum dose to evaluate if the ordered dose is a safe dose.
   2. **167.99 mcg is the maximum dose for a child who weighs 42 lbs. The ordered dose is 150 mcg, therefore the ordered dose is a safe dose.**
   3. 83.99 mcg is the minimum dose for a child who weighs 42 lbs. The nurse needs to calculate the maximum dose to evaluate if the ordered dose is a safe dose. The ordered dose is a safe dose.
   4. 167.99 mcg is the maximum dose for a child who weighs 42 lbs. The ordered dose is 150 mcg (less than the maximum dose), therefore, the ordered dose is a safe dose.

Module Test 5 (con't)

8. **Option 2. 17 gtt / mL**
   Rationales:
   1. This flow rate is not correct. The hourly rate is 83 mL / hr and the drop factor is 12 gtt / mL.
   2. **This flow rate is correct to deliver 83 mL / hr.**
   3. This flow rate is not correct. The hourly rate is 83 mL / hr and the drop factor is 12 gtt / mL.
   4. This flow rate is not correct. The hourly rate is 83 mL / hr and the drop factor is 12 gtt / mL.

9. **Option 1. The maximum dose is 20 mg. This is an unsafe dose.**
   Rationales:
   1. **This is correct. The maximum dose is 20 mg. The ordered dose is 25 mg. Therefore, the ordered dose is not a safe dose for this patient.**
   2. The maximum dose is 20 mg. The patient weighs 80 kg. 80 kg multiplied by 0.25 mg / kg equals 20 mg. The ordered dose is not a safe dose for this patient.
   3. The maximum dose is 20 mg. The patient weighs 80 kg. 80 kg multiplied by 0.25 mg / kg equals 20 mg. The ordered dose is not a safe dose for this patient.
   4. 28 mg is the maximum dose if the nurse uses 0.35 mg / kg for a repeat dose. The physician's order is for an initial dose of diltiazem.

10. **Option 3. Use a U-50 insulin (1/2 cc) syringe to administer the Humulin NPH insulin.**
    Rationales:
    1. A tuberculin (16 minims) syringe is not a correct choice of syringe to measure insulin.
    2. A U-100 insulin (1 cc) syringe is calibrated to measure even numbered doses. Therefore, it cannot accurately measure 21 units.
    3. **A U-50 insulin (1/2 cc) syringe is calibrated to measure odd-numbered and even-numbered doses. Therefore, this is the best syringe to use to measure the ordered dose.**
    4. The 3 mL syringe cannot accurately measure insulin doses and should not be used to administer insulin.

Appendix

Body Surface Area Nomograms for Children

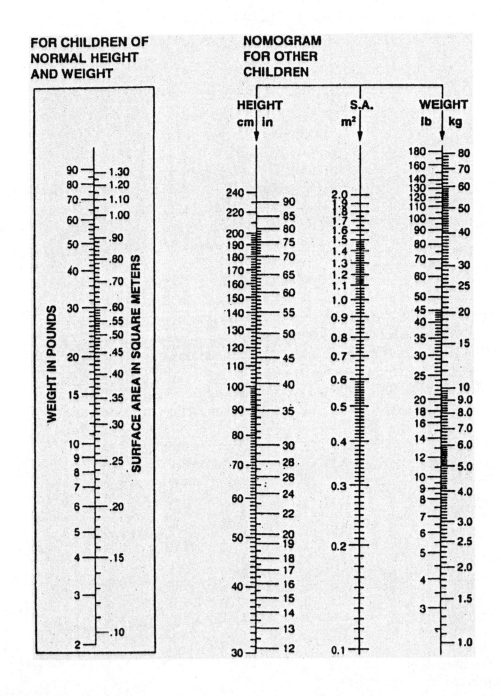

(In Behrman RE, Vaughan VC, eds. *Nelson Textbook of Pediatrics*, 16th ed. Philadelphia, PA: WB Saunders Co., 2000.)

Appendix

High Alert Medications

While most medications given by nurses in the clinical area have some possibility of risk for the patient, some medications have a greater potential for harm than others do.

The Institute of Safe Medication Practices (ISMP) has identified a list of high alert medications that require extra care and safeguards. These medications can cause serious injury or death if improperly ordered, prepared, stocked, dispensed, administered, or monitored. These medications may be dangerous due to a narrow therapeutic range, or an inherently toxic nature. The Joint Commission on Accreditation of Healthcare Organizations (JCAHO) monitors the five most frequently prescribed high alert medications: insulin, opiates and narcotics, injectable potassium chloride (or phosphate) concentrate, intravenous anticoagulants, and sodium chloride solutions above 0.9 percent.

The second edition of *Calculating Drug Doses: An Interactive Approach to Learning Nursing Math* includes a new focus on the high alert medications. A new section called High Alert Medications (with pertinent safety information and related nursing implications) is included in each module in the CD. More safety-related information is included in the Student Workbook and Instructor's Guide.

The following is a list of high alert medications found in the second edition of *Calculating Drug Doses: An Interactive Approach to Learning Nursing Math*:

amiodarone
bleomycin
busulfan
carmustine
chlorambucil
codeine
colchicine
dacarbazine
daunorubicin
digoxin
dobutamine
dopamine
droperidol
epinephrine
eptifibatide
esmolol
fentanyl
floxuridine
gemcitabine
heparin
heparins (low-molecular
    weight/heparinoids)

hydrocodone
hydromorphone
insulins (asparte, glargine,
    lente, lispro, NPH,
    regular, concentrated
    regular, ultralente)
labetalol
lidocaine
magnesium sulfate
meperidine
methadone
metoprolol
midazolam
milrinone
morphine
norepinephrine
potassium supplements
propranolol
sodium chloride
vinblastine
vincristine
warfarin